Birth

YOUR WAY

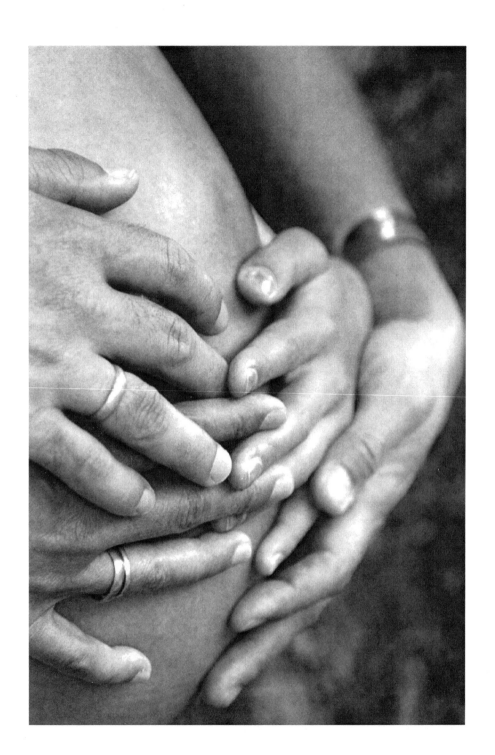

Birth
YOUR WAY

— Choosing birth at home or in a birth centre —

Sheila Kitzinger

with photos by Patti Ramos

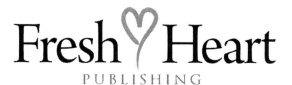

Fresh ♥ Heart
PUBLISHING

3rd British edition with references

1st edition published in 1991, 2nd in 2002, by Dorling Kindersley

This revised, updated and redesigned edition published in 2011 by
FRESH HEART PUBLISHING
a division of Fresh Heart Ltd
PO Box 225, Chester le Street, DH3 9BQ, United Kingdom
www.freshheartpublishing.co.uk

A CIP catalogue record for this publication is available from the British Library

ISBN: 978 1 906619 18 3

Set in Franklin Gothic Book, Eras ITC and Bradley Hand ITC
Designed and typeset by Fresh Heart Publishing
This English edition is an updated, adapted version of the original text
Fresh Heart Books for Better Birth series editor: Sylvie Donna
Printed in the UK by Lightning Source UK Ltd
Cover design by Fresh Heart Publishing
Cover photo of Tess McKenney with her home birth baby, Sam, by Uwe Kitzinger
All other photos by Patti Ramos, except those on pages 1, 8, 103, 112, 127,
159, 161, 174, 175, 198, 199, 216, 258, 277 and 333

Disclaimer

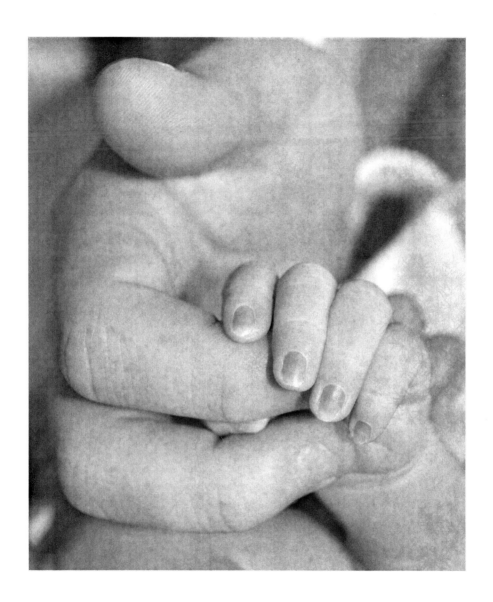

Dedication

Dedicated to those mothers and midwives who share
the experience of birth with understanding and joy—
and to my daughter Tess, with gratitude for her skills
and wisdom on which I have depended in revising this book

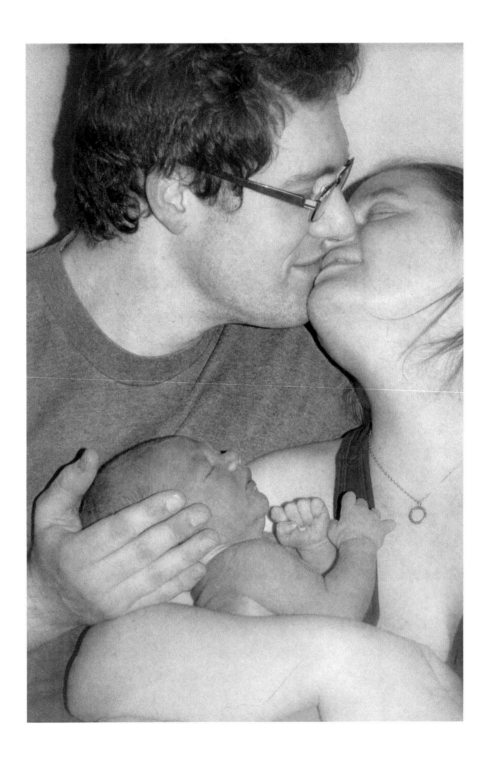

Contents

Making arrangements 84

Your midwife   112

Getting ready   128

Breathing your baby out... Tuning into your baby...
The power of touch...

Your birth partner   176

Sharing the experience   202

Meeting challenges   216

Enjoying your babymoon 258

Acknowledgements

I would like to thank my many friends and colleagues in the birth movement internationally who have explored with me different aspects of the subject of birth at home and in birth centres, and the social anthropologist the late Dr Margaret Mead who gave me strong encouragement to study birth in different cultures when she contributed to anthropological seminars in Oxford.

My daughter, Tess McKenney, who is my website designer and manager, and has had three home births in water, also works with me, giving information and support to women who seek choice in childbirth. My thanks also to Rachel Clark, Lorna Munroe, Michele Dodd and more recently Sue Allen, who achieved the mammoth task of sorting out all the references, have provided invaluable secretarial assistance. This book could never have been written without all the women who have discussed with me their own birth experiences, good and bad, from whom I have learnt a great deal.

I have absorbed so much from mothers, midwives, obstetricians, sociologists, psychologists, doulas and human rights activists in countries around the world that I feel I bear a precious burden of responsibility to convey this to every woman who opens these pages. I would also like to honour every woman who dares to assert her rights to challenge a powerful technological medical system and come to her own informed decisions.

Sheila Kitzinger

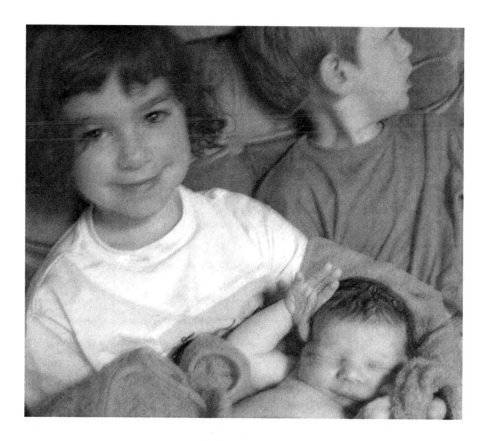

Why give birth at home or in a birth centre?

Having a baby is one of the most important passages in your life. You feel the child develop and move inside you. In labour you swim with contractions that are like tidal waves sweeping through your body. As you push the baby down, you know the intensity of the birth passion, and then reach out with eager hands to welcome your baby and cradle this new life in your arms. To see love made flesh is to witness a miracle.

BIRTH CHOICES

Whether birth is difficult or easy, painful or pain-free, long and drawn-out or brief, it need not be a medical event. It should never be conducted as if it were no more than a tooth extraction. For childbirth has much deeper significance than the removal of a baby like a decayed molar from a woman's body. The dawning of consciousness in a human being who is opening his or her eyes for the first time on our world is packed with meaning for the mother and father, and can be also for everyone who shares in this greatest adventure of all.

At least, that's how many women see birth. Not all of us, of course. There are women who think too much fuss is made about the birth experience, who simply want it to be painless and over with as soon as possible so that they can get on with their lives. That is a valid point of view. Some women are happy to accept induction, an epidural, and a forceps delivery, or a planned caesarean section, and they feel more secure knowing that childbirth is being managed by a top obstetrician with skills that augment or replace the natural process.

There are many other women, however, who want to have the information that will enable them to make their own decisions and to prepare themselves for an experience in which they participate fully. They know that it is easier to do this on their own ground, in a place to which the doctors and midwives come as guests. They would like to give birth outside hospital. This may be either in their own home, or in a birth centre in which the rhythms of a labouring woman's body are honoured and waited on, and where birth is non-interventionist and centred on people instead of on mechanical processes.

Hospitals exist where all members of staff share this attitude, but they are few and far between. You need only one person who is out of tune with such ideas, who believes in the aggressive management of labour, who, instead of being client-oriented, sees a woman as a patient who must obey hospital protocols, one person who is anxious and afraid, and who cannot trust women's bodies, for the environment in which birth takes place to be poisoned, and become completely unsuitable for the focused concentration and inner confidence that is needed for a good birth.

I believe that women should be able to have what they choose in childbirth. It is our bodies to which this is happening, and other people should not make decisions for us or make us feel guilty because they would have chosen a different way.

What is a 'good birth'?

A good birth is not just a matter of safety, or of achieving the goal of a live and physically healthy mother and baby. We want birth to be as safe as we can make it, but should not take it for granted that delivery in an operating theatre is necessarily the best way to achieve this. Childbirth has to do with emotions as well as with the sheer mechanics of descent, rotation and delivery. It is bound to be so, because childbirth is a major transition in the life of the mother, the father, and the whole family.

Childbirth has to do with emotions as well as sheer mechanics

Everything that happens in birth influences the way in which a woman perceives herself afterwards. It can affect the relationship between her and the baby, and between both parents and their baby, for years to come. Women have written to me to seek help with their intensely negative feelings about births that occurred 30 or 40 years earlier, in an attempt to exorcise finally the self-hatred, guilt and alienation that they experienced from then on.

A good birth is one which the woman looks back on, whatever happened, with satisfaction and fulfilment. Birth can be a positive experience even when, for reasons that cannot be avoided, there is a great deal of pain, or sometimes grieving. I have known a woman labour with a baby who she knew had already died. She was nurtured by her partner's loving support and, mingled with the agony of loss, there was an awareness that the experience was tender, compassionate and profound.

Women who give birth at home believe that home offers the best environment for themselves and their babies. It is far from being a selfish or thoughtless choice. Working towards this kind of birth, and often struggling for it, entails much self-searching, questioning and negotiation.

66 They helped me wrap him up in soft winceyette. He cried a bit. He wasn't particularly interested in the breast but gave it the occasional lick. Then Nick held him while they delivered the placenta without need of syntometrine. It slithered out five minutes after the birth.

Reasons for choosing birth at home or in a birth centre

Time and again, in discussions I have had with women about their reasons for choosing to give birth at home or in a birth centre, rather than in a hospital, the same priorities emerge. If you choose to give birth at home or in a birth centre, your reasons may also be...

♥ To have a relaxed, peaceful atmosphere for labour and birth.

♥ To feel the security and comfort of a familiar environment.

♥ To know that you are free to be yourself, to do whatever you feel like doing, to move around as you wish, to give birth in any position you choose, and to make any noises that come spontaneously.

♥ To have no interventions, either high-tech obstetric ones, or others that are often done routinely in hospitals, such as artificial rupture of the membranes.

♥ To be able to labour without drugs, and to explore other ways of handling pain.

♥ To know that those caring for you are your guests rather than managers, and that they make decisions together, instead of decisions being imposed on you.

♥ To enjoy a relationship of equality with those caring for you.

♥ To have a 'midwife birth' rather than an 'obstetric delivery'.

♥ To share intimately with others who are close to you; to enjoy the feeling of a loving community.

♥ To keep the family together; have other children there or close by.

♥ To avoid an episiotomy and perhaps achieve an intact perineum.

♥ Never to be separated from your baby.

♥ To be cared for after the birth in a way that is personal and intimate.

Women who choose home birth often have the same priorities

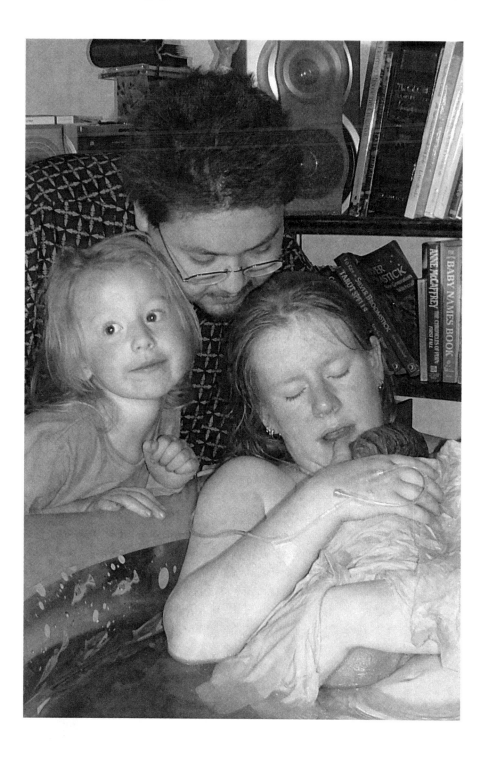

Women who retain control and understand the options available to them are much more likely to experience birth as satisfying

❝ It's the difference between nurses rushing past you in the corridor, in a place where you don't belong, and inviting people into your home, the place that belongs to you.

Women who feel that they can retain control over what is happening to them during the birth, who understand the options available, who are consulted about what they prefer, are much more likely to experience birth as satisfying than those who are merely at the receiving end of care, however kindly that care is. When birth is disempowering, a woman feels degraded, abused and mutilated. But when birth is empowering, the experience is enriching, her self-confidence is enhanced and she has a sense of triumph, however difficult the labour was.

When birth is empowering, the experience is enriching

I studied women's experiences of epidurals [1-7] and found that women who felt free from any pressure to have one, who were able to obtain the information they wanted and could share in decision-making, were more likely to feel positive about the birth than those who were under pressure to have an epidural and who felt deprived of autonomy in childbirth. As one woman put it: "I was helpless, treated like a side of meat, moved, examined, and catherised without consultation as though my labour now belonged to the doctors." In contrast, women for whom the decision to accept the offer of an epidural was an expression of their autonomy in childbirth, rather than a consequence of powerlessness and despair, have said, "I felt in control," or "I felt marvellous. I had gone from feeling and behaving like a caged wild animal to being myself, a rational human being." So a central issue in women's birth experiences is that of control: whether we can maintain control over what happens to our bodies, or whether control is taken from us.

❝ In the first hour after birth a baby is alert and responsive, so is much more interesting to meet than a bundle in a cot.

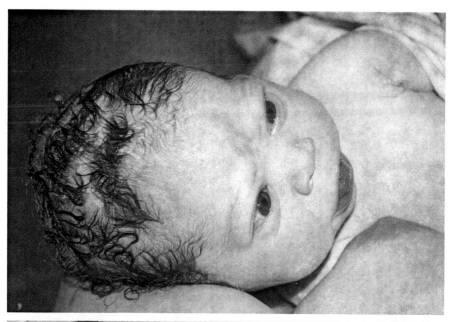

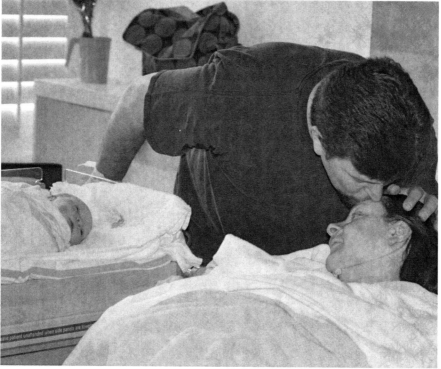

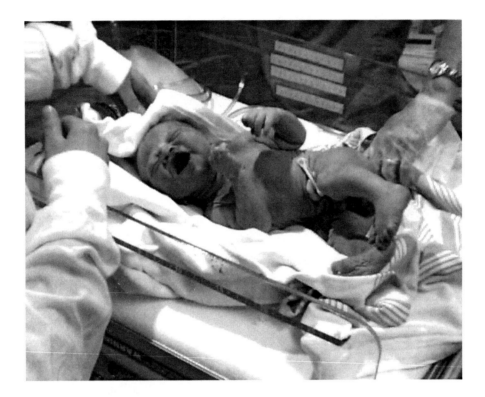

Questioning hospital practices

One reason why you may be considering birth outside hospital is that you have heard from other women about their unhappy experiences, have visited the hospital and did not like the atmosphere, or have already had a hospital birth and are determined not to repeat the experience. The same hospital that offers superb care to people who are ill may provide an environment for childbirth that introduces unnecessary risks, obstructs the normal process, and inculcates in women who are giving birth anxiety, dependency, fear, and loss of self-confidence.

THE HOSPITAL SYSTEM

The maternity hospitals of the 18th and 19th centuries were created as charity institutions for poor women who had nowhere else to go and for unmarried women bearing their babies in shame. (Other women gave birth at home.) These institutions provided raw material for obstetric practice, and women were used to demonstrate obstetrics and gynaecology to medical students. They were guinea pigs for research too. The first experiments for artificially inducing labour were conducted on poor women who could not afford doctors' fees and who entered hospital as clinic patients.

In the United States poor women without health insurance still provide a pool of patients on whom students can learn. In Britain women having babies in teaching hospitals may also find medical students grouped round the bed, and they may never discover that the doctor who laboriously stitched an episiotomy was a house officer learning how to do it for the first time.

Following the Second World War, the British National Health Service made medical care accessible to all without need to worry about payment. Many other European countries created social security and health care systems funded by tax payers, based on the policy that health care is a national responsibility.

With the creation of the National Health Service there came government health policies about childbirth and where it should take place. The decision was made that there should be sufficient beds for all women to have their babies in hospital, and birth became more and more medicalised. This was happening at a time when the standard of living was rising fast. A generation of British children had grown up who had benefited from the simple, good nutrition of the war years—wholemeal bread, orange juice, milk, relatively little fat, little meat, and high consumption of vegetables. People were healthier than ever before. As a result women were more likely to be fit during pregnancy, they did not suffer from anaemia, and did not think of pregnancy as an illness. Babies were born healthier, and the perinatal mortality rate—the number of babies who die at birth or soon after—dropped progressively, until it was 8 per 1,000.

With the creation of the NHS there came government health policies about childbirth and where it should take place

*Still today, women at the bottom of the social scale
are twice as likely to have a baby who dies*

Obstetricians claim that this improvement was due to better obstetric services, and to the policy of hospital birth for all. Yet still today women who are at the bottom of the social scale, whose partners are manual workers or who are unemployed, are twice as likely to have a baby who dies as middle class women. Social differences—education, general health, access to information, housing conditions, nutrition, attitudes to smoking, and ease of communication between caregivers and patients—have a powerful effect on the perinatal mortality rate (babies who die at birth or soon afterwards). Babies die and women suffer in childbirth and afterwards because of poverty and neglect.

Sophisticated equipment, modern, high-technology machines, anaesthetists and doctors with surgical skills are available only in hospital, of course. This equipment and these skills can be life-saving for a small minority of babies. But increasingly researchers are asking whether the intervention that takes place, often routinely, in many hospital births may not be hazardous. Most techniques have been introduced without adequate research. The question is whether procedures such as induction of labour, stimulation of the uterus with drugs once labour has started, artificial rupture of the membranes, the use of large quantities of pain-killing drugs, and continuous electronic monitoring of the fetus may not be harmful for mothers and babies if they take place as a matter of routine and are not used selectively.

Hospital ritual

The trouble is that almost every woman going into hospital today finds that procedures she does not wish to have are mandatory because of hospital protocols about care and rules laid down by obstetricians. Many interventions occur...

- Your waters are sometimes broken artificially when your cervix is 3—4cm dilated.

- If your cervix does not dilate by 1cm per hour your labour may be speeded up. This entails an intravenous drip in your arm and a uterine stimulant dripped into your bloodstream.

- You may be under pressure to have drugs for pain relief that you don't want.

- You may be allowed only two hours, or an hour and a half, or an hour, or even 45 minutes, to deliver following full dilation—before being given a forceps delivery or vacuum extraction because 'the baby is at risk'.

There are more subtle interventions too, things that affect the atmosphere in which birth takes place and the attitudes of everyone participating. They include:

- Having to put on a hospital gown

- Being put to bed as if you were ill

- Not being able to eat and drink when you want to

- Constant checking of the progress of labour against the clock

- Different members of staff coming and going

- Having no privacy and being surrounded by strangers who talk over you and about you, rather than to you

- Being treated like an irresponsible child who is not given any control

In some hospitals the whole emphasis is on pathology—detecting things that might go wrong—instead of on supporting the spontaneous flow of labour.

These interventions can lead to a massive loss of confidence in a woman. She is expected to be passive and obedient, a 'good patient'. She comes to distrust her body. She may feel alienated from everything that is happening to her, even though caregivers are trying to be kind. They may be unaware of how she is feeling and of the distress that is bottled up inside her, to emerge only later, days, weeks or months after the baby is born. She is likely to believe that all her negative emotions about the birth and the way in which it is replayed over and over again in her mind, and sometimes too, the hostility that bursts through towards her baby, are her own fault, and she feels terribly guilty.

66 They just told me what they were going to do. They never asked what I wanted.

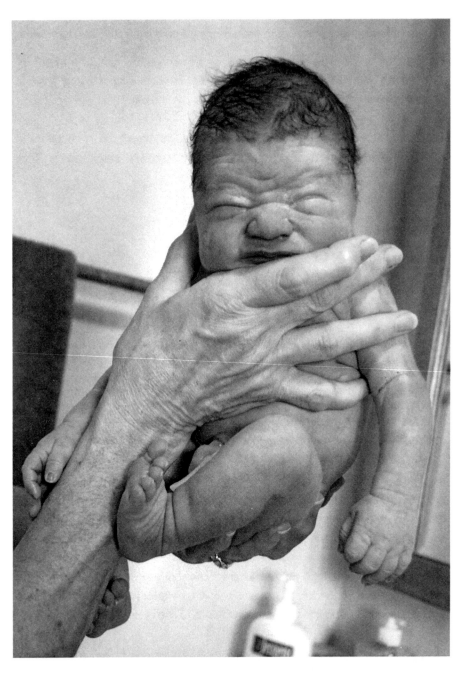

The trouble is that almost every woman going into hospital today
finds that procedures she does not wish to have are mandatory
because of hospital protocols about care

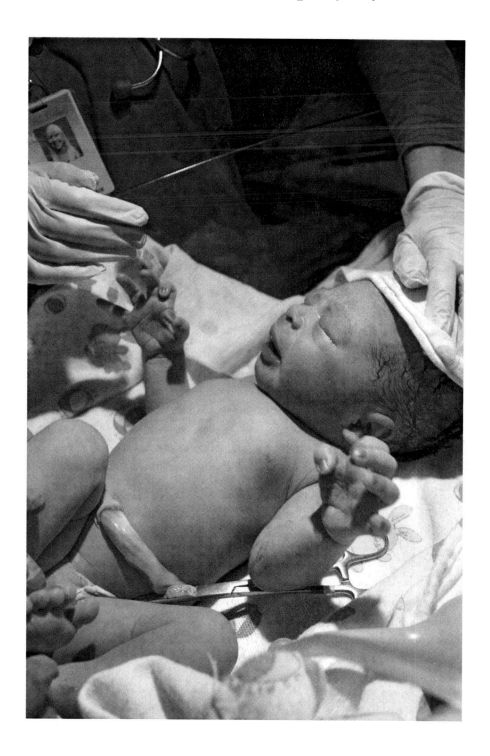

New developments

Astonishing changes in obstetrics and in women's attitudes to childbirth occurred from the 70s and up to the present day. A new partnership between obstetrics and electronic engineering opened up windows on the womb with ultrasound; technological innovations made birth more complicated, compelling the mother to be a passive patient; and birth was seen by obstetricians as a medical event that could take place only in an intensive care setting equipped to meet all possible disasters. At the same time, women have been clamouring for care that is more personal, more sensitive to their needs, in an environment in which they can be in tune with the spontaneous psycho-biological processes of birth and with the creative energy pouring through their bodies.

66 It isn't a matter of what it looks like. The hospital birthing rooms are all chintzy. But the staff decide what you do and when you do it. They're in control. I don't want to be 'managed' by anybody.

The result has been, on the one hand, more and more obstetric intervention and, on the other, a reformation movement in which women are rediscovering the value of small-scale, low-tech birth places, seeking alternative settings such as birth centres and birth rooms, and even, in spite of intense opposition from the medical system, making the decision to give birth in their own homes.

A woman describing her home birth:

66 Birth is birth, not pain. Closing my eyes I can imagine the birth of mountains to describe the forces at work in my body.

Women walk about throughout the first stage of labour and midwives—and more rarely obstetricians—allow mothers to be in any position which is comfortable for them to give birth. Birth plans are sometimes used. Women are asked what they would like, and caregivers are listening more to their patients, and recording their wishes in the case notes. All this is to be warmly welcomed. We are making progress.

66 *One question to resolve is, "Will birth in this place be both safe and empowering for me as a woman?"*

Even so, hospitals are institutions, and often very large, complex, bureaucratic, and hierarchically organised institutions. They have to be managed so that the different parts of the whole structure can work together efficiently. Under these circumstances it is easy to abrogate responsibility and for an individual's main concern to be to oil the wheels of the system and make it run smoothly. It is not surprising that women's needs and wishes are often ignored or trivialised. Hospitals would function much more efficiently if there were no patients.

In hospital patients may be allowed choice, but they have no real power. The territory belongs to the hospital management. When I analysed the words and phrases used by 40 women who had given birth at home and compared their accounts with 40 others spoken by women who all delivered vaginally in hospital, I found that many of those in hospital used words such as 'allowed' or 'let me', but no home birth mothers used these words. Although many hospital birth mothers felt very positive about their experience, they did not have the same sense of being able to control what happened to them.

66 *Breathing slowly, feeling the pain with satisfaction and pleasure, in my own room, at peace...*

Pain is never as simple as just having a 'high' or 'low' pain threshold. Pain always has a meaning. It does not exist in a vacuum. It rouses personal memories of being in pain and witnessing other people's pain. The way we approach pain may be affected by other women's descriptions of their labours, as well as by birth images in books and the media, and often half-forgotten childhood memories, too.

The way we approach pain may be affected by other women's descriptions of their labours, as well as by birth images in books and the media, and often half-forgotten childhood memories too

How do you usually handle pain? Not only labour pain, but other kinds. If you immediately reach for some capsules to deaden it, home birth may not be right for you. If you think about what *causes* the pain, and as a result try to reduce the pressures you are under, if you change what you eat, adjust your posture and the way you move, and especially if you have discovered how relaxation, breathing and focused concentration can help you handle pain, home birth may be a good choice. Home birth works best for women who want to *cope* with pain rather than hand the pain over to be reduced or eradicated by professionals.

❝ The head crowned and stayed as the contraction went off and whoa! What a stretch! I had to pant as I waited for the next contraction and wondered if I would split open! Bobbie passed me a mirror and I shook my head, trying to stay focused. Then quickly my body gave another push and out came the head.

Labour pain is different from the pain of injury. It is caused by muscles stretching, pressure against nerves, and the body opening. It is similar to menstrual pain, but much more intense. It comes in waves. This rhythm means that there is a rest period between each contraction. As your cervix dilates progressively these rest periods become very short. There is just time to breathe out, drop shoulders, relax, and centre yourself, before the next wave rushes over you.

The *meaning* of birth pain is different from the pain of, say tooth or earache, broken bones or colic. It is the pain of creative activity. In a labour that is going well each contraction starts gently, builds up in a grand crescendo to a peak, and then fades away. It is pain with a purpose—*positive* pain.

This is not to say that birth pain is easy to bear. For many women it is the hardest pain they have ever experienced. It has been rated among the most severe pain ever known. Yet it is profoundly affected by what is going on in your mind and the attitudes of whoever is helping you.

Pain is a private experience. No-one can tell you that their pain is more or less than yours. This is why it is difficult to evaluate and place it on a scale of 0 - 10. It all depends on the significance that the pain has in terms of your life, your relationships and the surroundings.

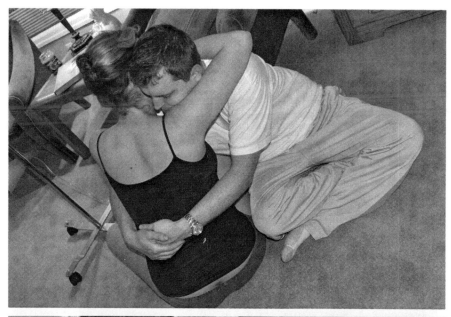

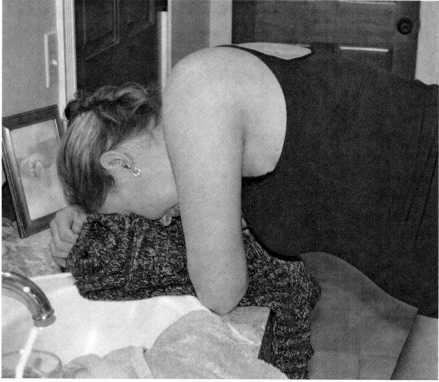

> ❝ I looked down to see her on the floor, a wriggling, slithering little body with all her rolls of loose skin, pale and brown stained, hair plastered onto her head. I said, 'Hello, my darling, it's OK' and put my hands down to pick her up.

It is difficult for anyone who has had a distressing labour to understand how other women can enjoy giving birth. It seems to some women that when others talk about the joy of birth and of triumphantly riding the waves of contractions they must be romanticising or telling lies. A woman who, for example, relies on getting an epidural as soon as she turns up at the hospital but is denied one because the anaesthetist is not available, or the midwife considers it too late in labour to give it and that it would lead to an unnecessary operative delivery, is likely to feel extreme and uncontrollable pain. She also feels anger that may be turned on to those who denied her pain relief and other women who look back on their labours with satisfaction and delight. It is not hard to understand why this happens. It does not rule out the fact that it is possible to relish the birth experience in the right environment with the right people. For those who choose home birth, being on their own territory is an important part of this.

> ❝ I had just climbed Annapurna and accepted the Nobel prize all in the course of little more than a day.

Research reveals that women who are not looking forward to the baby suffer more pain than those who are eager to have the baby. When a partner is negative about or hostile to a pregnancy this may lead to birth being more painful too.[1, 2]

When a woman is very anxious towards the end of pregnancy she tends to feel more pain in labour than one who is happy, and if she *expects* to feel a lot of pain, she really experiences more, probably because she is tense and already in a state of psycho-physiological 'fight or flight'.[3] And when a woman is isolated and alone during the first stage of labour everything becomes more painful.[4]

When a woman is very anxious, she tends to feel more pain than one who is happy. If she expects to experience a lot of pain, she usually experiences more, probably because she's tense.

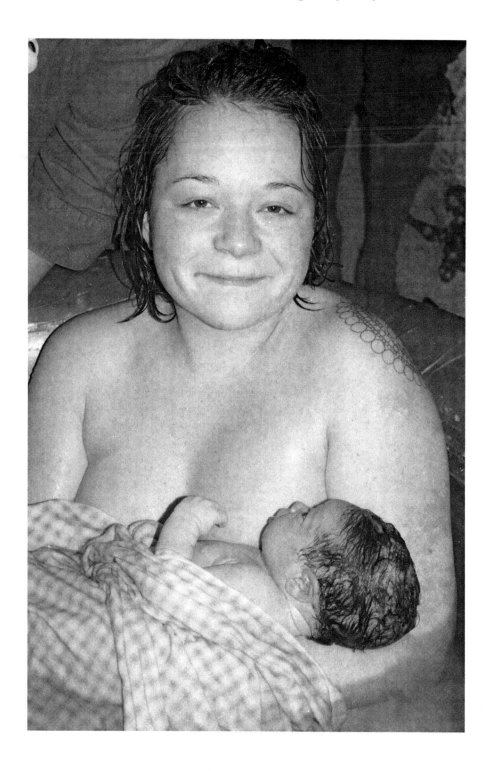

The effects of stress

Labour is stressful for most women, even in an out-of-hospital setting where they feel safe, confident, and among friends. In hospital, environmental stress is added to this psychological stress.

Hospital birth is often very stressful because a woman is in a strange place, she has to cope with a number of different professionals who care for her, and the emphasis is on things that may go wrong. It is not simply a matter of pain. This added stress combines with the stress from the pain. Distress tends to interfere with the efficiency of uterine action, and labour slows down or she is unable to push her baby out. Because it interferes with the physiology of birth, this excessive stress may affect the condition of the baby before and after birth.

> 66 She was so slippery and I was now shaking uncontrollably so Bobbie helped her into my arms and I lay back and held her on my tummy. I could hardly hold her for shaking and her squirming and slipperiness, but there she was, and I was trying to calm us both.

When under stress our bodies produce catecholamines, or 'stress hormones', the best-known of which are adrenaline and noradrenaline. This is normal and advantageous under most circumstances, because catecholamines help the body adjust to stress. If the stress is excessive, however, or goes on for too long, the body exhausts its resources and can no longer adjust to the stress.

When catecholamine levels rise abnormally in a woman in labour her uterus contracts less efficiently, contractions become weaker or spasmodic, dilation of the cervix is slower, and labour takes longer.[5] Sometimes the uterus simply stops contracting for a while. This often occurs when a woman first arrives in hospital, even when contractions have been strong and regular at home. The rise in catecholamine levels has the effect of making her more anxious, which also means that she feels more pain. This in turn further increases catecholamine levels. It is a vicious circle.

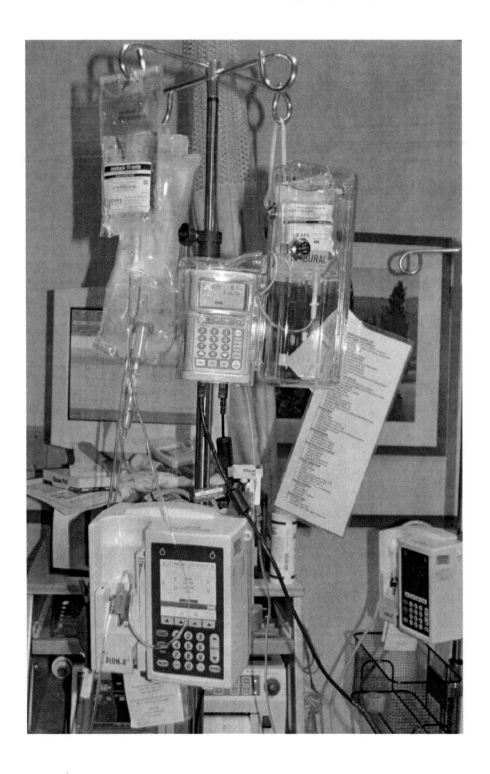

When there's no added stress contractions are good for the baby

However, when there is no added stress, the hard work of labour, the mother's excitement, the mobilisation of her energy to meet the challenge of contractions as they get stronger, longer, and closer together, are good for the baby. The fetus also makes its own catecholamines. When catecholamines are at a normal level, they:

♥ Push up production of prostaglandins and stimulate oxygen uptake

♥ Protect the baby from the effects of reduced flow of blood through the placenta at the height of contractions

♥ Cause blood to be shunted from near the skin surface to the baby's vital organs—the heart, brain and liver—and energy stores are mobilised ready for birth

They help the baby adjust to life outside the uterus by:

♥ Facilitating absorption of liquid in the lungs

♥ Enabling the baby to generate its own heat

♥ Producing the alert, attentive state that helps parents fall in love with their baby

66 Though stinging, trembling and in shock, I was ecstatic. I couldn't believe it. Here was that being I'd been talking to all those months, longing to hold in my arms. I gave thanks for our safe delivery and whispered, 'We did it. We're safe. I love you.'

A doctor:

66 I have just had my first baby at home. It was an incredible experience—the equivalent of climbing Mount Everest.

Having my baby at home was an incredible experience

But catecholamines are pushed above this physiological level when the mother is under great stress during labour. When this happens...

- Less oxygen-ated blood flows to the uterus and through the placenta to the baby.

- The baby compensates by increasing its own production of catecholamines to excessive levels, with resulting fetal heart irregularities due to lack of oxygen.

Very high catecholamine levels may lead to problems for the newborn baby too. These include:

- breathing difficulties

- difficulty in regulating his temperature so that he becomes very cold

- reduction in plasma volume (the liquid part of blood)

- metabolic acidosis (disturbance in the chemical balance of blood)

- jaundice (excess bile pigment in blood)

- even sometimes necrotising enterocolitis (diarrhoea with blood in the faeces)

> The hospital environment, with its rules, tests, and constant threat of obstetric intervention, pushes up both the labouring woman's catecholamine levels and also those of her baby

Obstetric anaesthetists who are concerned about the effect of high catecholamine levels on babies respond by recommending that small hospitals should be closed, all women moved to large regional hospitals and as many offered epidural anaesthesia as the epidural service can handle.[6] An epidural can provide blessed relief when a woman is in uncontrollable pain. But often the pain is actually caused or made uncontrollable by the way she is being treated. The hospital environment, with its rules, tests, and constant threat of obstetric intervention, is pushing up both her catecholamine levels and those of her baby.

WHY NOT HOSPITAL?

Hospitals are often dangerous places in which to give birth. It is usually taken for granted that they must be safe because they have the equipment and skilled staff to deal with medical emergencies. But sometimes they are the cause of these emergencies in the first place. Many interventions that take place routinely in hospital birth are iatrogenic. That is, they result in illness produced by doctors.

An obstetrician:

66 When a woman is at home and you want to intervene, it forces you to think whether it's really necessary. The very ease with which interventions take place in hospital increases the risk of them being performed unnecessarily.

Induction

The most frequent reason for women to be transferred from home to hospital before labour starts is to be induced.

The artificial start of labour, induction, is done in one, or a combination, of three ways:

- Synthetic oxytocin is introduced into the woman's bloodstream.

- Prostaglandin in the form of a gel is placed in the cervix.

- Amniotomy is performed—the water bubble in which the baby lies is broken with an instrument resembling a crochet hook, or with small forceps.

Rates of induction vary widely in different countries, and between different obstetricians. Women often do not even know why their labours are being induced. It is the doctor's decision, and the mother is expected to go along with it for the sake of her baby.

Women often don't know why their labours are being induced

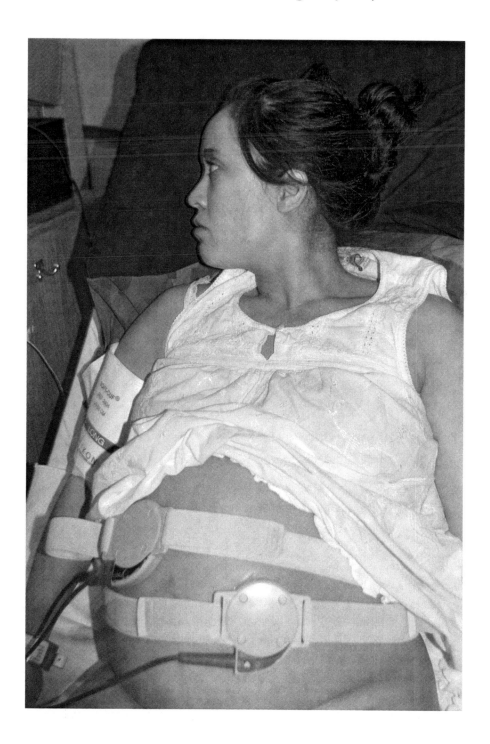

A doctor may want to induce if a woman goes two weeks, ten days, or even a few days, past her due date. Some like to induce at term—on or around the expected date—on the grounds that 'this is a very precious baby', especially with an older mother. There are women who prefer to know exactly when the birth will be. These inductions for convenience are often disguised as medically indicated.

Induction, like other interventions, can be useful in selected situations: if a woman has pre-eclampsia, for example, and her blood pressure is dangerously high, the placenta may fail to support the baby, and it may be safer to deliver early. A diabetic woman's baby tends to grow very large and, though premature, may be more safely delivered early.

But induction is not always successful. It is most likely to succeed if a woman's cervix is ripe. Ripeness is assessed by the 'Bishop score'. Only if that exceeds 8 are the chances of success the same as if labour starts spontaneously.

66 The pain was shocking—double-peaked contractions that lasted almost two minutes.

The risks of induction

Induction does not always work.[7] Failed induction leads to caesarean section.

- If the baby's head is not well down and membranes are ruptured artificially the first rush of amniotic fluid may bring the cord down and deprive the baby of oxygen.

- Artificial rupture of the membranes can cause infection.

- An induced labour is often fast and furious, so is more painful than one that starts naturally. In my own study of some women's experiences of induced labour[8] I found that when women whose second labour was induced compared this in retrospect with the previous labour which had not been induced, two-thirds of them said that the second labour was more painful, although as a rule second labours are less painful.

- Because induction is often given in a package deal with epidural anaesthesia, other interventions may take place which add new risks with a knock-on effect. Having a catheter inserted in the bladder increases the risk of infection, for example. Being immobilised makes it more likely that dilation is slow, and so the drip is turned up and more artificial oxytocin (syntocinon) is fed into the bloodstream. Large quantities of fluid may produce water intoxication. A woman who drinks as much fluid as she wants during labour does not take too much. But if fluids are introduced through an intravenous drip her metabolism is altered and if she receives an excessive quantity, she may suffer convulsions. When synthetic oxytocin is being dripped into a woman's bloodstream in addition to glucose solution, she is further at risk of water intoxication.

> Because induction is often given in a package deal with epidural anaesthesia, other interventions may take place which add new risks with a knock-on effect

- Occasionally the uterus becomes hypertonic—it clamps down on the baby with strong contractions lasting two minutes or longer—and this reduces the flow of blood. In normal labour contractions squeeze the baby as if it were being hugged tightly. Blood flow is lessened at the height of contractions but increased as each one finishes. In induced labour there is a risk that this rhythm is lost and that the uterus goes into spasm. The result is that the baby's heartbeat becomes either very fast (tachycardia) or slow (bradycardia). At birth the baby may need resuscitation and be taken to the special care nursery for observation.

> In induced labour there is a risk that the rhythm of labour is lost and that the uterus goes into spasm

- Hyperstimulation of the uterus sometimes results in uterine rupture, especially in women who have had babies before, and those who have had a caesarean.

- There is increased risk of amniotic fluid embolism—a bubble of fluid entering the mother's circulation.

- It is impossible to move freely, or sometimes even to change position in bed with ease. The woman has little bits of plastic, wire, and rubber sticking out all over her: an intravenous drip in her arm; a blood pressure cuff encircling her upper arm; a catheter in her bladder; an electrode screwed or clipped into the baby's scalp to record its heartbeat; and a plastic tube stuck in her back and snaking up to her shoulder, where it is fixed with sticky tape so that the epidural can be topped up.

- Because labour is always monitored electronically when induction takes place, warning signs in the baby's heart rate are watched for. A worrying print-out may unfurl from the monitor, there may be flashing red lights, and alarm bells may be triggered. This is distressing for a woman in labour.

- The chance of an operative vaginal delivery or a caesarean is increased. The operative vaginal birth rate (forceps or ventouse) goes up by 1.5 (half as much again) and caesareans by 1.8 (almost twice as many are performed), even when induction gets labour going.

At home or in a birth centre labour is not induced, for it is recognised that induction brings risks and may entail other forms of intervention, including drugs for pain relief and an assisted delivery, which are incompatible with care outside hospital. Having a baby at home is one way of ruling out entirely a whole category of risks that starts with induction, escalates with pain-killing drugs, and peaks when uterine stimulants are stepped up because drugs have made contractions weaker or erratic.

Induction Q&A:

Q: Why are labours induced?

A: Inductions, like other interventions, can be useful in selected situations. If a woman has pre-eclampsia, for example, and her blood pressure is dangerously high, the placenta may fail to support the baby, so it may be safer to deliver early. A diabetic woman's baby tends to grow very large and, though preterm, it might be safer to deliver early.

Q: Are there any other reasons?

A: A doctor may want to induce if you go two weeks, ten days, or even a few days past her due date. Some like to induce at term—on or around the expected date, or even a week early—on the grounds that 'this is a very precious baby', especially with an older mother. There are women who are fed up with being pregnant or who prefer to know exactly when the birth will be, and who welcome induction for this reason. Inductions for convenience are often disguised as medically indicated.

Q: How is labour induced?

A: Induction is done in one, or a combination, of three ways: synthetic oxytocin is introduced into your bloodstream. Prostaglandin in the form of a gel is placed in your cervix. Amniotomy is performed—the water bubble in which the baby lies is broken with an instrument resembling a crochet hook, or with small forceps.

Q: Will I still be able to have an active birth?

A: No. It is impossible to move freely, or sometimes even to change position in bed with ease. You have an intravenous drip in your arm, a blood pressure cuff encircling your upper arm, a catheter in your bladder, an electrode screwed or clipped into the baby's scalp to record its heartbeat, and if you have an epidural, a plastic tube stuck in your back and snaking up to your shoulder, where it is fixed with sticky tape so that the epidural can be topped up.

Q: What other interventions might there be?

A: Because induction makes labour more painful it is often given in a package deal with epidural anaesthesia. Then other interventions may take place which add new risks with a knock-on effect. Having a catheter inserted in your bladder increases the risk of infection, for example. Labour is always monitored electronically when induction takes place. This increases the chance of an operative vaginal delivery or a caesarean.

Having a catheter inserted increases the risk of infection

Active management

In many hospitals today labours are managed 'actively'. The obstetrician takes charge, with the aim of making labour conform to a norm. A typical pattern is that it should not last longer than 12 hours, dilation should take place by at least 1cm an hour, and delivery must occur within one hour of full dilation.

> In many hospitals today labours are managed 'actively'—
> the obstetrician takes charge, with the aim of
> making labour conform to a norm.

If a labour is not conforming to this model, intravenous synthetic oxytocin is used to stimulate the uterus to greater activity, or delivery is completed with forceps, vacuum extraction (ventouse), or caesarean section.[9]

> A woman is told at noon that her baby is expected at four o'clock

Active management was first introduced in Dublin, where the emphasis was on a short, snappy labour, and also on one-to-one nurse care. (For some reason the Irish obstetricians who started this system ignored midwives and talked about 'nurses' instead.) They called it 'military efficiency with a human face'.[10] The original plan was that fathers should be present, epidurals would be given and pethidine available in small doses. "The time of delivery is stated to within 30 minutes: a woman is told at noon that her baby is expected at 4 o'clock in the afternoon, give or take half an hour."[11] Women must labour silently: "A woman owes it to herself, to her husband, and to her child, and to every other woman who may be unfortunate enough to labour at the same time, to be well-briefed in this matter. The disruptive effect of one disorganised and frightened woman in a delivery unit extends far beyond her own comfort and safety, and there should be no hesitation in telling her so."

> 66 They ruptured my membranes, set up a glucose drip, and put a scalp electrode on the baby's head. I felt trapped. Then they added syntocinon to the drip and gave me pethidine.

> "The disruptive effect of one disorganised and frightened woman in a delivery unit extends far beyond her own comfort and safety"

According to these obstetricians, others have a duty also to those who care for them during labour: "It should be clearly understood that nurses must not be expected to submit to the sometimes outrageous conduct of perfectly healthy women who cannot be persuaded to ... behave with dignity and purpose during the most important hours of their lives—nor should nurses be held responsible in any way for the degrading scenes which occasionally result."[12] So, when a woman pleaded for pain-killers, wept in terror, or screamed out in agony, these obstetricians considered it her fault.

" I had an intravenous drip and was strapped up to two fetal monitors. I longed to get upright, but it was impossible.

The use of oxytocin to augment labour is not without risk

The use of oxytocin to augment labour is not without risk. Just as when it is used for induction, labour is more painful for the mother, there may be hyperstimulation of the uterus, and the baby may become short of oxygen. This is why obstetricians in Dublin do not advise the use of oxytocin in multigravidae (women who have already had babies). Elsewhere, however, active management may include the routine speeding up of labour, even when the problem is not, in fact, uterine 'inefficiency' but disproportion—that is, when the baby cannot pass through the mother's pelvis. Then the uterus may rupture (the muscle tears), and the baby may be squeezed so hard and often that there is shortage of oxygen (hypoxia); in some cases the baby may turn out to have cerebral palsy as a result, and the mother's pelvis may even be fractured.[13]

" I was given [synthetic] oxytocin with no explanation. They told my husband, "She's being a bit slow." It was a very shocking experience.

When you give birth in territory which you control, instead of management protocols dictating how labour should be conducted, you are yourself the active birth-giver. This is the fundamental difference between birth in hospital and birth at home or in the kind of birth centre where the power is yours, not the doctor's.

Electronic fetal monitoring

Many obstetricians believe that continuous electronic fetal monitoring should be employed in all labours 'just in case'. In hospital, monitoring is done either from the time a woman is admitted until she delivers, or a 'strip' print-out is taken for about an hour after she is admitted and, if all is well, taken again only if further information is required later on in the labour.

There is marked disagreement between obstetricians about what ought to be done when the print-out from the monitor is different from what would normally be expected. When four experienced obstetricians studied the same fetal heart traces and were asked whether they would deliver immediately, they agreed in only one out of five cases.[14] Nearly two years later these obstetricians were shown the same traces again and asked what they would do. In one out of five cases they assessed them differently from the time before.

There is no evidence that electronic fetal monitoring saves babies' lives or that the condition of babies at birth has anything to do with whether or not they had it during labour.[15] It has been discovered, however, that when babies are monitored they are less likely to have neonatal seizures.[16] This might be a very important finding except that further studies have revealed that these seizures are not linked with any long-term problems.[17]

66 They put me on an oxytocin drip against my will. I was left with a student who read the paper and totally ignored me.

Risks of electronic monitoring

At first glance it might look as if this particular piece of high technology could do nothing but good. But the trouble is that electronic fetal monitoring itself causes problems and introduces its own risks.

• If monitoring is to be employed safely, caregivers must know how to use it and understand how to interpret the information correctly. This is not always the case. Sometimes the monitor picks up the mother's heartbeat rather than the baby's, for example. Since the baby's heart is normally about twice as fast as the labouring woman's, it then appears as if there is fetal bradycardia. Unnecessary intervention takes place, and the baby may be delivered by forceps or caesarean section.[18]

- Sometimes the opposite happens: caregivers are lulled into a false sense of security when a woman is wired up to a monitor and no one bothers to check the print-out regularly or looks at the whole pattern of her labour. The monitor cannot give birth. Only the woman can do that. The monitor records data, and what is done or not done then depends on the skills of the caregivers.

- Although some monitors work with radio waves—telemetry—and allow a woman to walk about, the use of most monitors means that the woman must stay in one place, either strapped up tightly with belts around her abdomen or wired up with a pin stuck in the baby's head. This immobilisation causes unnecessary pain and may slow down contractions and make them weaker, so that dilation is slower. Sometimes labour becomes so slow that the decision is made to augment it with a synthetic oxytocin (syntocinon) intravenous drip.

- A woman is often told to lie still so that the print-out is clear.[19] If she is lying on her back, not only does she get backache, but there is a danger of compression of her vena cava—the large blood vessel in the lower part of her body—by her heavy uterus, with a resulting slow down in the flow of blood back to her heart. She becomes sick, dizzy, faint, and may even black out. This deprives the baby of oxygen too. The monitor then spills out ominous traces in the fetal heart rate, recording information about a situation which it was responsible for creating in the first place.

- When there are staff shortages, or when staff do not understand the importance of being centred on the woman and creating a calm, loving atmosphere, a partner is often told to keep an eye on the monitor, or a nurse or midwife pops in at intervals, studies the print-out, says a cheery word to the mother, and disappears again. Attention turns to the electronic equipment rather than being focused on the woman's needs and she loses emotional support. Even with her partner close beside her, a woman may then be emotionally isolated. An electronic monitor cannot take the place of human caring and understanding. Mind and body are not two separate, distinct systems in childbirth. A woman's body works best when she feels confident, secure, emotionally supported, and on her own ground.

66 Everything was just 'done' to me. I wasn't consulted about anything and it was all out of my control.

- An electrode can be fixed on the baby's head only after the membranes have ruptured. If this has not occurred spontaneously in early labour, an amniotomy is performed, usually at 3cm or 4cm dilation. When there is no interference, membranes usually do not rupture at the beginning of labour, but at the very end of the first stage. Artificial rupture of the membranes interferes with the sterile environment in which the baby is contained and may result in infection. It also removes the protection provided by the water bubble which normally cushions the baby and its cord and placenta against excessive pressure, so that blood flow is impeded. The monitor may then demonstrate that the baby is in trouble, but it was the amniotomy performed in order to put the electrode on the baby's head that was responsible for the stress to the baby.

- Some doctors are experimenting with ways of fixing electrodes using strong suction or glue so that they do not have to harpoon the baby, but they have not yet succeeded in producing a viable alternative to scalp clips or screws. When a baby's scalp is penetrated by the hook or spiral screw, there is danger of damage when removing it.[20] Sometimes there is a bald patch and hair never grows there, or a scalp abscess forms, which has to be treated with antibiotics.[21]

- In most hospitals the introduction of electronic fetal monitoring immediately pushes the caesarean section rate up at least three-fold. After the equipment has been in use for some time, staff relax a bit and the rate drops again. But in industrialised countries worldwide there is a steady rise in the caesarean section rate, which can be attributed partly to electronic monitoring. Caesarean section is riskier for women than vaginal birth. Five times as many women die after a caesarean section than after a vaginal birth (50 compared with 10 per 100,000 deliveries), and there is a much increased risk of infection and other postnatal problems.[22]

- Information from the monitor bears little relation to the baby's condition at birth. We don't know enough about normal variations in the heart rate to warrant intervention only on the basis of a suspicious trace.

Information from the monitor bears little relation to the baby's condition at birth. We don't know enough about normal variations.

- Many monitors don't work well all the time. Women say that they were told: "Oh, don't take any notice of that. It isn't working properly," or a husband is advised to kick the machine when a light starts flashing because "It's always doing that. It doesn't mean anything." Yet the rule is that the woman must be attached to a monitor, even though it is not providing accurate information. This can be a very bewildering and frightening experience. Under these circumstances the monitor is worse than useless. It is dangerous.

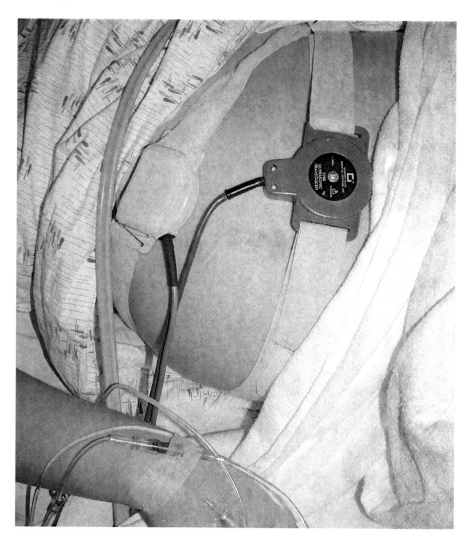

Intermittent monitoring

The older way of monitoring the condition of the baby during labour was to listen to its heart intermittently through a trumpet-shaped fetal stethoscope. The accuracy of this method depends on how often and when it is done. It is important to know whether the fetal heart is picking up regularly after contractions. The baby who is over-stressed is usually the one whose heart speeds up a lot—above 160 beats a minute—or slows down below 120 beats a minute with contractions, and stays high or low in the space between contractions. When the heart slows down at the peak of contractions, a perfectly natural occurrence, it is called a Type 1 dip. When the heart stays slow afterwards, it is a Type 2 dip. It is the Type 2 dips that are worrying. If a baby is in real trouble, there are few or no variations in heart rate. The trace is flat. So if a fetal stethoscope is the method of choice, it should be used at the end of every cluster of strong contractions in the late first stage, and more often in the second stage, the times in labour when contractions may be most stressful for the baby.

Having a fetal stethoscope poked at you just as a contraction ends can be uncomfortable and irritating. Many women and midwives prefer a newer intermittent method of monitoring which uses Doppler ultrasound in the form of a hand-held Sonicaid. This is a camera-sized instrument with a disc like a small microphone which is held over the baby's heart, registers the beats, and translates these into an audible signal—like galloping horses.

This method provides no permanent record of the heart rate in the form of a printed trace, and this could be a disadvantage from the point of view of obstetricians anxious about possible litigation after the birth. However, litigation is very unlikely after a birth that has taken place, by the woman's choice, out of hospital without obstetric intervention.

So high-tech gadgets may be useful, but only those that do not intrude on your ability to tune into your own body and to the power that wells up inside you, on the full tide of which your baby is brought to birth.

The only gadgets which are useful are those that don't intrude on your ability to tune into your own body—to the power inside you

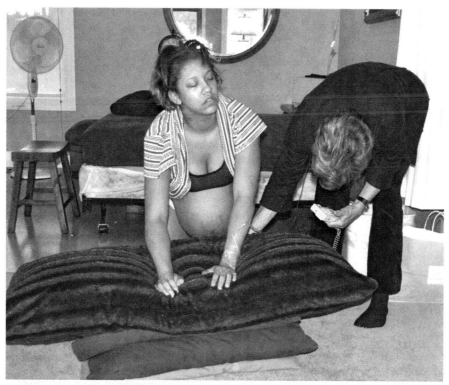

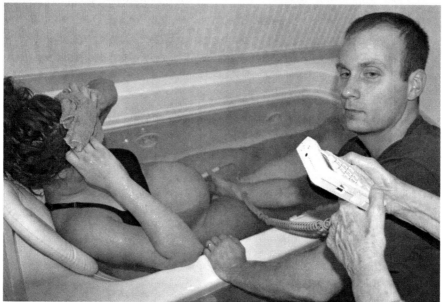

A doctor:

66 I did a home birth and had for the first time a feeling of confidence because it was just happening. Any medical intervention would have been entirely inappropriate.

Pain-relieving drugs

One reason why women seek home birth is that they hope to have a drug-free labour. All anaesthetic and analgesic drugs given to the mother cross the placenta to the fetus. I have heard an obstetric anaesthetist describe the placenta as 'a sump for drugs'. Drug transfer is flow dependent. Fetal plasma has a lower pH than maternal plasma, so the drug concentrates in the fetus. Pethidine, for example, is a weak analgesic but a strong respiratory depressant. After a single dose there is a higher concentration in the fetus than in the mother, and it can be detected in the newborn baby for 62 hours.

Epidurals

An epidural can give blessed relief from pain and it does not produce respiratory depression. When performed by an experienced anaesthetist it is usually safe. But it may have side-effects for the mother and the baby. 15% of mothers and babies develop fever during labour. The baby may be taken to the special care nursery for investigation and tests to discover if it is suffering from septicaemia.

The mother's blood pressure may drop suddenly when the epidural is given and this reduces the oxygen through the placenta passing to the baby. So other drugs have to be available to raise her blood pressure again. Delivery may be by forceps or ventouse (vacuum extraction) because the tone of the pelvic floor muscles is lost, the head gets stuck in the wrong position, and she cannot push the baby out. The vaginal operative delivery rate is four times higher than when a woman does not have an epidural, and the caesarean rate is twice as high. Paralysis is extremely rare.[23]

The vaginal operative delivery rate is four times higher

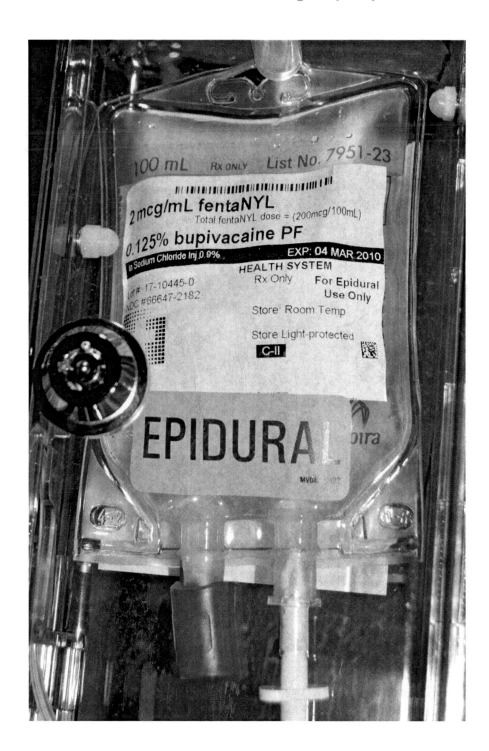

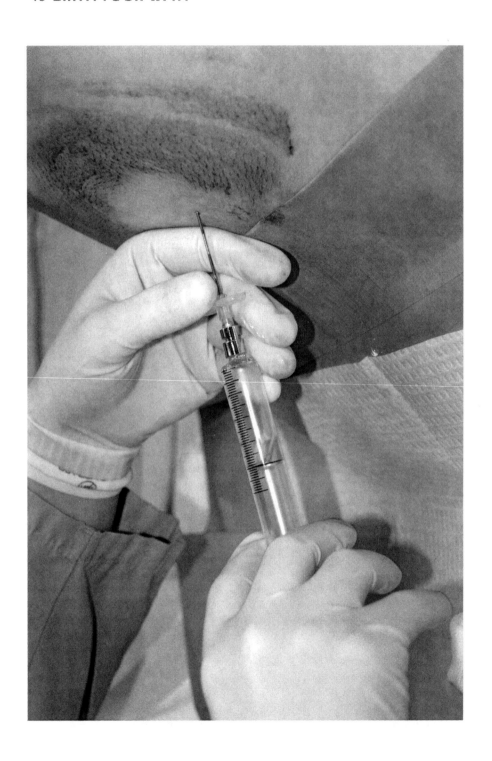

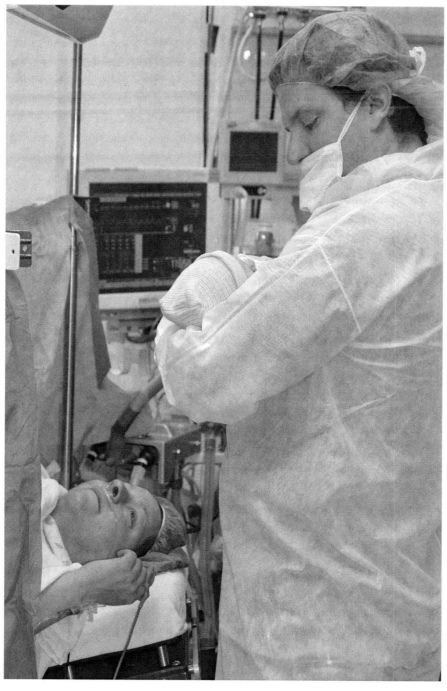

The rushed second stage

Clock-watched labours are the rule in hospitals. When women describe their labours in hospital, they often refer to the time and say things like: "My induction was well-timed to fit into working hours," "The pupil midwife told me to watch the clock and time contractions," or "The baby was posterior, and the midwife said they'd give me a few hours to see what happened." When women give birth at home, they talk about mealtimes, sunrise, sunlight pouring through the window, sunset and night time, but they do not usually relate everything that occurred in labour to the clock.

In my own study of the language women used in describing 40 home and 40 hospital births, three-quarters of home birth mothers said that they enjoyed not being hurried and knowing that they had plenty of time.[24] Only four hospital birth mothers made similar statements.

In hospital the clock is master, marking the distinction between the normal and the abnormal, the labour that can be allowed to proceed without obstetric intervention and the one that calls for immediate intervention.

Doctors and midwives who attend home births usually know how to watch and wait. They realise that the uterus works most effectively if a woman is in an upright or semi-upright position and can alter her position when she wants. They know that moving around can often change malposition or mal-presentation. They are aware that anxiety and fear can make it harder for a woman to open her body and push her baby out. If she is not wasting energy trying to push and pushes only when she wants to, and for only as long as she wants to, she can work with her body, instead of fighting against it.

❝ The doctor gave me 20 minutes to push while she got the forceps ready. It was harrowing.

A second stage in which you are harried and hurried is bound to be an anxious and panic-inducing ordeal. In hospital women are often coaxed or commanded to push, and instructed to hold each breath and push as hard as they possibly can, because of the time limit on the second stage.

A second stage in which you are hurried is bound to be anxious

In British hospitals women having their first babies (primiparae) usually are allowed only one hour from full dilation to delivery. Some obstetricians consider that this is far too long, and limit first-time mothers to 45 minutes or even half an hour, and multiparae (women who've given birth before) to 20 minutes.[25]

There is no evidence that reducing the length of the second stage makes labour any safer, prevents baby deaths, or produces healthier babies.[26] If a baby is too large to come through the mother's pelvis, there are many clinical signs, including the head staying high, lack of progress, fetal heart arrhythmia, or Type 2 dips that indicate this—not the length of the second stage alone.

The fact that the mother is often encouraged to hold her breath over prolonged periods when pushing can be dangerous, because it may reduce the baby's oxygen.[27] One problem in many hospitals is that the second stage is reckoned to start with full dilation of the cervix. Frequent vaginal examinations result in full dilation being assessed and noted on the case record or partogram (labour chart) immediately it is reached, or even sometimes before this. The second stage is then timed from that point. But the woman may not yet want to push. This is natural. If the baby's head is not pressing against your pelvic floor muscles, you have no spontaneous desire to push, since this is a reflex stimulated when there is pressure against nerve endings in the pelvic floor. From that moment it is a race to the finishing post. The woman may be bullied in an effort to get the baby born before the obstetrician must be called, and delivery is usually completed with episiotomy and forceps or vacuum extraction, or a caesarean section.

Episiotomy

You are much more likely to have an episiotomy—a cut in the vagina to enlarge the birth opening—if you have your baby in hospital than if you give birth at home or in a birth centre. Episiotomy rates vary widely between countries, and even between hospitals and different obstetricians in the same hospital. In some countries nine out of ten women receive an episiotomy.[28] Some obstetricians believe that all first-time mothers should have an episiotomy. They may believe, too, that any woman who has had an episiotomy should have one with the next delivery, because scar tissue must be present that will not stretch to let the baby out easily. The result is that everyone has an episiotomy except those who deliver too fast to have one.

Pros and cons of episiotomy

Episiotomy is performed with the aim of saving the baby from being 'battered' against the mother's pelvic floor, to prevent damage to these muscles, to avoid injury to her anus, to prevent later stress incontinence (leaking of urine), and to achieve better healing than after laceration with 'a nice clean cut that is easier to sew up than a nasty, jagged tear'. There is no evidence that episiotomy does any of these things.[29] Even if it did not matter what happened to the mother and if episiotomies were performed for the baby's sake alone, the claim that episiotomy protects the baby's head or produces a baby in better condition is not supported by the evidence.[30]

Because obstetricians make rules as to how long their patients may be in the second stage, midwives and junior doctors delivering babies with no obstetrician present perform episiotomies to hasten delivery if they come up against that time limit.[31]

Although occasionally the baby's head can be nicked by scissors, the hazards of episiotomy generally concern the mother, not the baby, in a number of ways:

- Having an episiotomy is often acutely painful. If it is performed at the height of a contraction when the perineum is stretched and bulging, a woman may not feel it. But, because of possible damage to the baby's head, in hospitals there are rules about it being done only between contractions. A local anaesthetic is often—not always—given first, but this itself hurts in a very sensitive place, and in many hospitals staff do not wait the three or four minutes necessary for the perineum to become fully numb before cutting.[32]

Having an episiotomy is often acutely painful

- Repair of an episiotomy is often painful, too. The wound must be sutured carefully, correctly aligning damaged tissues. Inadequate local anaesthesia may be used, or an area is not numbed at all, or the person doing the suturing may not wait for the anaesthetic to take effect. So perineal repair is for some women more painful than anything they experienced during the birth—much more painful than contractions or the delivery.

- The area is often bruised. This may be because the baby's head has been bumping against it, but the most severe bruising results from an episiotomy made too early, before the head is on the perineum. This is regular practice in some hospitals, on the grounds that in this way any stress caused by the baby's head is prevented. The scissors used may be blunt, so that they crush as well as cut the tissues, and extensive bruising results then, too.

- Blood loss with episiotomy may cause anaemia and make a woman feel very weak and tired, and this at a time when she wants to be alert to get to know her baby. The combination of exhaustion and pain is demoralising and makes a frightening start to motherhood.

- Many episiotomy wounds become infected, and sometimes a perineal abscess results. This is terribly painful. Infection is more common in hospital than at home, and many hospital bacteria are now penicillin resistant. Infection delays healing and, when the wound does at last heal, there may be scar tissue.

- Although episiotomies are performed on the theory that to make a deliberate cut prevents a tear into the anus and rectum (a third-degree laceration—fourth-degree in the USA), this occurs more often when an episiotomy has been performed than when a tear occurs naturally. A small proportion of women have an episiotomy plus a laceration, because the cut has then gone on to tear. The intricate embroidery that has to be done when this happens may entail general anaesthesia and can take a long time. The woman is in far more pain afterwards than after a second-degree laceration.

- In the week after a woman's perineum has been sutured, as healing takes place, she is likely to be in constant discomfort, and in acute pain when she empties her bladder or bowels, walks, shifts position in bed, or lifts and feeds her baby. Women on postnatal wards shuffle around, bent forward, knees together, trying to cope with this pain. The second, third, and fourth days are often the worst, and then things become easier. The pain after a first-degree tear—a nick in the skin only—is much less than that after an episiotomy, which corresponds to a second-degree tear, cutting into muscle.

The lasting effects

Pain often lasts for some months, with a knot of scar tissue at the lower end of the vagina which may be too painful to touch. At three months postpartum a large percentage of women still have pain some of the time: if they sit down on a hard chair without thinking, wear trousers that are tight on the crotch, stand too long, or move carelessly. Women whose periods have returned say that they cannot possibly use tampons. The reason for this is that suturing has been done too tightly, not allowing for the swelling that follows injury to tissue that is especially sensitive. If you have ever seen anyone with a wasp sting near the eye, you know how enormous the swelling is. Perineal tissue is similar.

After an episiotomy it is impossible to have intercourse until everything has healed. At three months more women who have had episiotomies have pain with attempted intercourse than do those who have had even severe tears. Those still in most pain are women who have had both an episiotomy and a tear. A woman who cannot bear the thought of love-making because she is in pain often feels that it must be her fault.

❝ My husband is very patient and understanding but he thinks I should be better by now.

A small proportion of women, even after painstaking suturing, are left with a recto-vaginal fistula (a gap in the wall between the rectum and vagina) and pass faeces through the vagina. So they have another operation weeks or months later for this to be repaired. The emotional as well as the physical effect of all this cannot be underestimated. They feel mutilated, abused, and dirty. They may feel scalding anger or be deeply depressed.

Some women have pain that continues for years. Sometimes this happens because the vagina is too tight, with the tissues stretched and aching. Sometimes nerves have been sliced through. Sometimes a large knob of scar tissue remains painful, and the woman feels as if she is sitting on thorns. When she seeks help, she may be advised to lubricate the painful area, be told that the pain will pass eventually, be sent to a psychotherapist or marriage counsellor, or be offered surgery to cut out scar tissue and improve the 'cosmetic' result.

In home births and birth centres episiotomies are not done automatically. They are reserved for those situations in which a baby needs to be born quickly. Midwives have skills of "guarding" the perineum with a hand, enabling a woman to give birth slowly and gently, so that the perineum is not over-stressed and there is less likelihood of a tear. They use hot compresses, warm water, or oil massage to soften tissues and help them to fan out, and often words that suggest vivid opening images.[33] Many also use new methods such as birth in water, which seems to help maintain the elasticity of a woman's perineum.

Drugs and infections in hospitals

Two major interrelated problems in hospitals today are cross-infection and resistance to antibiotics. At home a woman can usually cope with bacteria in her own family. Moreover, since she is not exposed to obstetric intervention at home, damage to tissue, whether on the surface of her body or deep inside it, is unlikely to allow the introduction of harmful bacteria. The baby is resistant to many infections, both because of immunity built up through the placenta while inside the uterus and from maternal colostrum and breast milk after birth.

> Two major interrelated problems in hospitals today are cross-infection and resistance to antibiotics

Pelvic, bladder, perineal and breast infections are normally treated with penicillin or related antibiotics. These are highly effective if used when a woman has a caesarean section (which brings with it an increased risk of pelvic infection as well as infection of the scar). But liberal use of penicillin produces resistant strains of disease. Bacteria are clever and adapt rapidly to threat. "In 1941, 10,000 units of penicillin administered four times a day for four days cured patients of pneumococcal pneumonia," a specialist at Columbia University writes.[34] He says that today the patient could have 24 million units a day and still die.

Hospitals started using antibiotics in the 1950s. Today approximately one patient in every three is on antibiotics. We do not know how long it will be before there are so many genetically modified, penicillin-resistant strains that penicillin becomes useless. Some doctors are already claiming that we face a global epidemic.[35]

Newborn babies as patients

In hospital the moment that babies are born, and even before birth, they are treated as patients, and subjected to a range of painful practices which cause distress and interfere with their smooth adjustment to life.

- In many hospitals the first assault on babies as they are born is to suction them, by passing a tube into the nose and mouth to extract any mucus that might be in the airways. This suctioning of the baby's nasal passages and throat is especially distressing for the baby when done roughly, using a catheter rather than a suction bulb.[36] It may result in cardiac arrhythmia and if the catheter touches the larynx, it is likely to cause laryngeal spasm. Occasionally the herpes virus or bacteria are transferred through the suction catheter to the baby from the midwife or doctor.[37] Even with babies who have already passed meconium (the first contents of the bowel)—a sign that they are under stress—it is uncertain whether intubation does more good than harm.

- In some hospitals another routine is to pass a tube down into the baby's stomach to clear any gastric secretions that may be there. This scouring of the baby's gastric tract is another assault. It leads to slowing of the heart rate and spasm of the larynx, which can interfere with the baby's whole pattern of sucking and swallowing—so that feeding is made more difficult.[38]

- Some countries have a law that all newborn babies must receive prophylaxis against gonorrhoeal blindness. This is not the case in the UK. Silver nitrate drops are put in the baby's eyes. They are intensely irritating and cause babies to close their eyes, interfering with communication between the mother and her baby in the hour following birth, the time when the baby is most likely to be in a quiet, alert state.[39] In fact erythromycin works better than silver nitrate[40] and is also effective against chlamydia, which a baby can pick up from the mother's vagina.[41] Silver nitrate is not effective against chlamydia.

In hospital you may have little or no control over what is put in your baby's eyes because there are often hospital protocols which do not permit choice. At home this is something you decide together with your midwife.

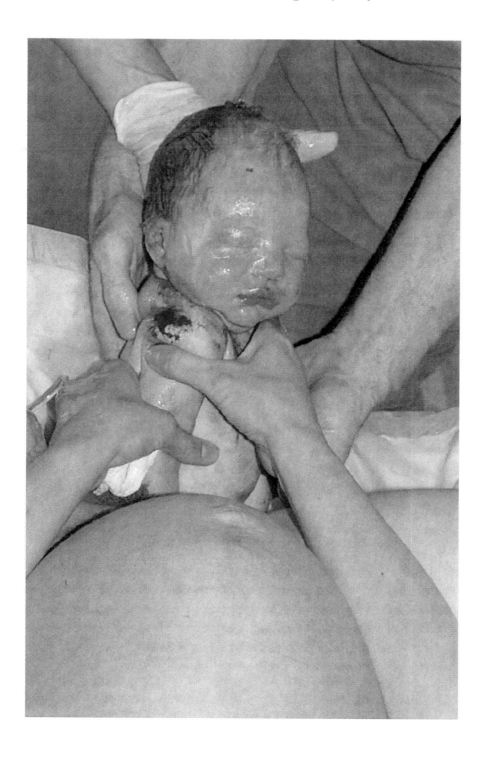

Tender, loving care?

In some hospitals large numbers of babies are moved to the special care nursery, if only for observation. In many countries babies are routinely separated from their mothers anyway, isolated in a small room with a large window where a nurse glances at them occasionally, as I have seen happening in Italy, or in a large nursery under bright, fluorescent lights with dozens of other babies, as in the USA, or even in a good-sized cupboard which nurses use as a refuge where they can chat and smoke—something that I saw in the former USSR.

When babies are herded together the risk of cross-infection is high and no one is likely to watch a newborn baby like its mother

Apart from the emotional deprivation caused to the mother by taking her baby away from her—the reward of all her work and striving—and the loneliness and confusion the baby may feel, this is bad practice. It can be dangerous. When babies are herded together in this way, the risk of cross-infection is high, and no one is likely to watch a newborn baby as unceasingly and with such acute observation as the mother.

66 Every part of me seemed to fill with what I can only describe as 'a loving ecstasy'. This intense communication was never possible in hospital immediately after birth, as the babies were not beside me. But I wonder if there it could have taken place. It was something so special I think it needed exactly the right receptive conditions on both our parts for it to happen.

Babies are treated as if they are the property of the hospital rather than the mother, and as if trained professionals are the only people who could safely assess a baby's condition and give appropriate care. When the World Health Organization enquired in 24 European countries what the usual practices were, it was revealed that in 17 countries babies were automatically separated from their mothers for a period of time after birth.[42]

In 27 countries babies were automatically separated from their mothers for a period of time after birth

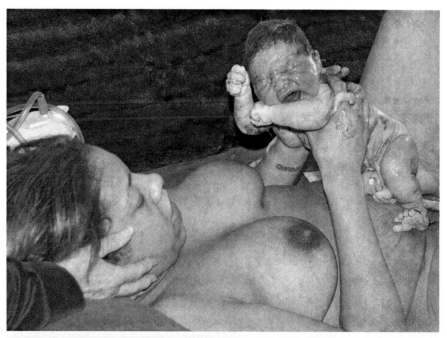

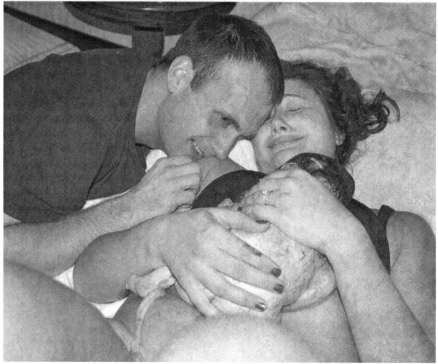

Bonding

Bonding is sometimes seen as something that must be 'facilitated' or actively taught by staff, rather than as a process that cannot be rushed, that occurs in its own way and its own sweet time if a mother has her baby with her whenever she wants, for as long as she wants, and if she is in a supportive, friendly environment.

In some hospitals bonding theory has been incorporated into care in very destructive ways. Women say they feel they have to put on a performance and respond to their babies in the correct, loving style, because they are aware that they are under the scrutiny of staff checking to see if bonding is taking place.

66 I knew they were watching me to see if we were bonding. But the birth had been such an ordeal I needed time. I couldn't be rushed. I felt I had to put on an act.

Being forced to take what amounts to an examination in motherhood within a few hours or even minutes of your baby's birth is not the best way of starting off a relationship. It interferes with the powerful emotions that may be sweeping through you and is likely to make you self-conscious, self-questioning and inhibited. Most women overcome these obstacles. But it is hard on those who have had a stressful and difficult birth and who may not be able to 'come back into themselves' and feel secure enough to reach out to their babies. They need peace and quiet, and to be nurtured themselves, before they can nurture their babies.

A GENTLER ALTERNATIVE

Many hospitals now practise 'gentle birth'. Lights are dimmed for delivery, voices hushed, the baby is handled gently and given to the mother immediately. She can cuddle her newborn against her bare skin under a special heater or a blanket which covers them both, and mother, father, and baby have uninterrupted time together for about an hour after delivery.

Many hospitals now practise 'gentle birth'. However…

Bonding is sometimes seen as something that must be 'facilitated' or actively taught, rather than as a process that cannot be rushed, that occurs in its own way, in its own time

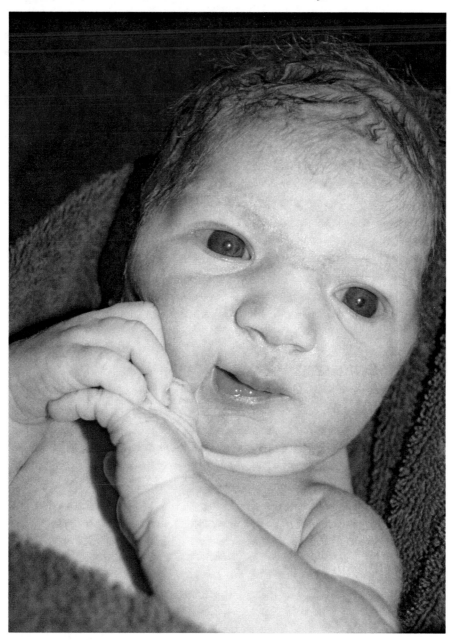

Most mothers don't realise that the baby may be taken
from them after the birth for a paediatric examination

So far, so good. But what mothers often don't realise is that the baby may then be taken from them to another place for a paediatric examination. This is a brightly lit, noisy nursery—a very different environment from the close intimacy of that first postnatal hour.

66 I want to spend time with the baby and my husband, talking about the whole experience and our feelings, without a time limit and without interference—in my own familiar surroundings.

At home, or in a birth centre your baby remains with you and will never be taken away from you for any reason whatever, unless you wish it. A woman watches her baby intently, fascinated by each tiny movement, listens to the strange and sometimes quick, dancing patterns of breathing. What is happening is important in the development of the relationship between mother and baby. To interfere with or destroy that intimacy is to risk interrupting a vital psychological process that may reduce the woman's confidence in herself as a mother and interfere with the flow of communication between her and her baby.

Another good reason to avoid hospitals...

You may decide on home birth to avoid a caesarean section. Having a baby in hospital increases the chance of an unnecessary caesarean. A major study of close on 50,000 women in south east England, which compared vaginal births with caesarean deliveries, reveals that those who had caesareans experienced four times as many life-threatening events, although there was no medical reason to expect any problems. These 'life-threatening events' included haemorrhage, infection and rupture of the uterus. (The researchers did not even start to estimate the risk of thrombo-embolism, which can result from surgery, because of difficulty in agreeing on the diagnosis.)[43]

You may decide on home birth to avoid a caesarean section.
Having a baby in hospital increases the chance of
an unnecessary caesarean.

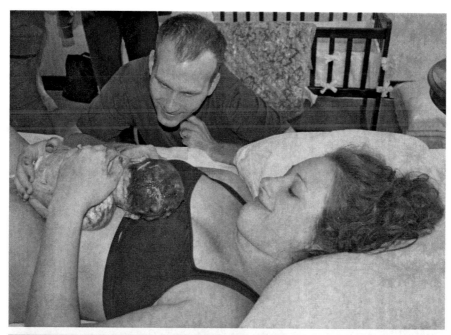

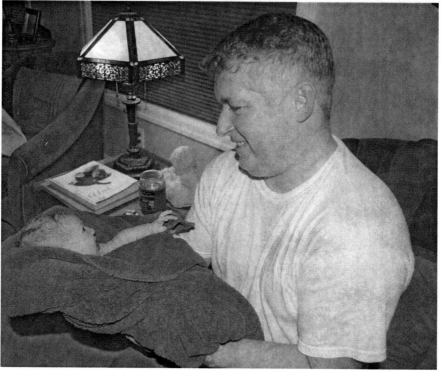

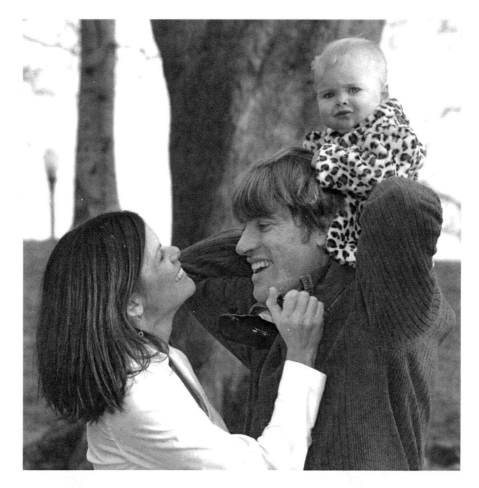

Understanding safety

Decisions about where to give birth should spring from realistic risk assessment and from your own values. Any woman who decides that birth without hospital is right for her in a society that is hostile to freedom in childbirth takes responsibility for weighing up risks. She also expresses the courage to resist autocracy, dogma and the power of the medical system. Her decision is based on deeply held values. Doctors, however, tend to see birth exclusively in terms of risk.

ASSESSING RISK

At your first antenatal visit the doctor may refer to a 'risk score' to decide which category of care is appropriate for you: ordinary doctor/midwife, care under the direction of obstetricians, or highly specialised and intensive care from an expert team. You may have little choice. You are labelled high or low risk either on the basis of a score like this, or simply because of the doctor's clinical hunches. With some risk scores, as many as nine out of ten women turn out to be 'high risk'.

❝❝ You are high risk because you are 31... It's your first baby and you have an untried pelvis... You had a miscarriage last year... You are in a high risk ethnic group... You are single... This is your fifth baby... Your last labour was induced and you had a forceps delivery... You have had a previous caesarean section.

Attaching labels to pregnant women is damaging. A woman assigned to a high risk category will probably have interventions that make birth more complicated, and women who are aware that they are 'at risk' lose confidence and become anxious. If everyone around you expects things to go wrong, you begin to believe that they will—and they may well do so.

❝❝ People say, "How brave you are, having your baby at home!" I don't feel brave at all. I think they're the brave ones, to go into hospital and risk all the things that are done to you there.

Often a woman is categorised as high or low risk without reference to her everyday life. Such things as poor housing, bad conditions in the workplace, little money for food, a violent partner, social isolation, unemployment, or family problems are social conditions which are at the roots of perinatal mortality (baby deaths) and morbidity (illness).

> Attaching labels to pregnant women is damaging.
> A woman assigned to a high risk category will probably
> have interventions that make birth more complicated.

It is not a matter of skin colour but of socio-economic conditions.

Assigning all black women to an 'at risk' category is racially discriminatory. There are wide variations in the lifestyles, economic circumstances, and the education of black women. Asian women who live in one area of London have no more baby deaths than the general population, whereas those in Bradford, in the north of England, are much more likely to suffer the death of a baby. It is not a matter of skin colour but of socio-economic conditions.

Sara Wickham, editor of *Essentially MIDIRS*, writes: "I suspect that many of us focus more on the concept of choice as it relates to discussion around invasive interventions ... than on the implications of risk assessment itself. Yet it is increasingly common that women are denied the right to birth in particular settings as a result of being deemed 'at risk', a label which may also lead to recommendation of further screening and/or prophylactic measures, each of which may again have emotional and social as well as physical implications."[1]

Birth, like all other human activities, is never entirely risk-free. But most risk markers used are very poor predictors and some are not evidence-based. Some doctors still believe, for example, that any woman with small feet must have a small pelvic outlet too, so may ask their patients what size shoes they wear, and those wearing Size 3 are automatically categorised as high risk. Research shows that this is ridiculous.[2]

Women often feel trapped with care that is imposed on them, which is very different from what they would have chosen themselves. To make decisions about the care we want and the place of birth, we need full and accurate information about potential risks and then we need to decide ourselves what to do. Some risk is acceptable. We may want to go on holiday, so we take a plane. We enjoy skiing or rock-climbing and accept the risk of a broken leg. The risks are worth it. If sailors worried about risk all the time, they would never go to sea.

We can also prepare to handle risks, taking sensible precautions against the most likely dangers. For example, we wear a life jacket on a sailing dinghy, or buckle on a seatbelt in the car, and we can learn what to do if risks build up.

We can prepare to handle risks, taking sensible precautions

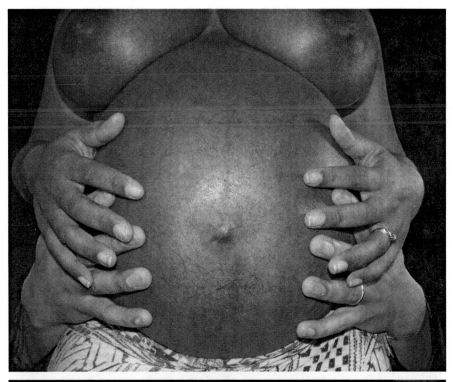

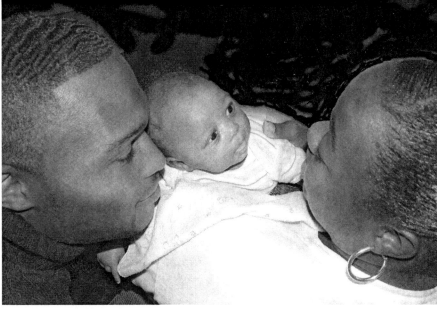

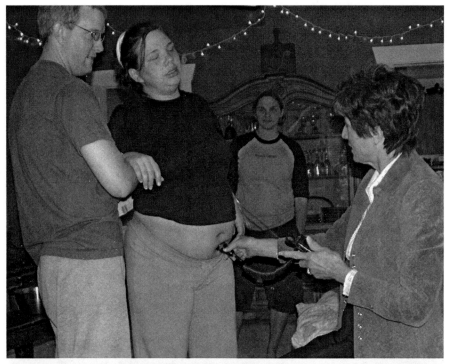

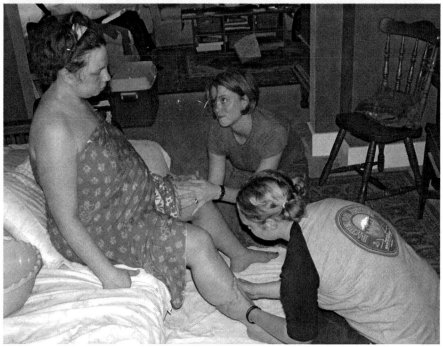

Risk Q&A for home birth:

Q: What equipment does the midwife carry?

A. The midwife will have simple equipment such as a Pinard stethoscope or a Sonicaid, some pain-relieving drugs, and other drugs to make the uterus contract after the baby is born if you bleed heavily. She may have aromatherapy oils, transcutaneous electronic nerve stimulation apparatus (TENS) to help you cope with pain, or a birth stool, or suggest that you get these things.

Q: What happens if the baby has breathing problems?

A: Babies are more likely to experience breathing difficulties if the mother has had pain-killing drugs in labour, especially pethidine or another opiate such as diamorphine. A woman may not have any drugs at all in a home birth. And if she does have pain-relieving drugs these are given in small doses. The midwife carries oxygen and simple resuscitation equipment is case it is needed.

Q: I had a caesarean before. Can I give birth at home this time?

A: It will be more difficult to get a doctor or midwife to agree. There are additional risks in having a baby outside hospital, but there are also risks with the unnecessary and harmful interventions that can occur in hospitals. It may be that the previous caesarean was the result of intervention, such as being induced, being stuck in bed, having an epidural, or fetal monitoring.

Q: I am very overweight. Should I have a home birth?

A: It helps to be within a normal weight range. But never go on a crash diet during pregnancy. This is bad for both you and your baby. Ask for help from a dietician.

Q: I am an 'older' first-time mum. Can I have a home birth?

A: Although your doctor may not be encouraging, if you are healthy and have a normal pregnancy, there is no reason why you should not plan a home birth, although there is a higher chance of being transferred to hospital during the first stage of labour simply because it may take a long time.

Minimising the risks

If you are going to have your baby at home, it makes sense to:

♥ Find a midwife you like. She should be skilled, confident, and relaxed in working in an out-of-hospital setting.

♥ Approach birth free from fear, self-assured and positive.

♥ Acquire the art of meeting contractions with relaxation, breathing and concentration, and learn about using different positions and movements.

♥ Have more than one birth attendant. Your caregivers need to work well together, and your midwife needs her own support. Think about having a doula, or birth companion.

♥ Ensure you have access to a telephone, and a car as well, if possible.

♥ Consider hiring a birthing pool.

Unravelling the statistics

It is often claimed that, because far fewer mothers and babies die than, say, 60 years ago, when most women had their babies at home, hospital birth must be the cause of improved survival rates. But the fact that two things happened at the same time does not mean that one caused the other.

Nor should we use statistics of home births from the past, or developing countries. Many other things are different, including our health, our access to contraceptives and abortion, and our socio-economic conditions. These have a profound effect on perinatal mortality. As the standard of living rises, fewer babies die at birth in every country, whether or not they are born in hospital.

Unplanned births outside hospital are often included in the statistics for home births, and this gives a completely wrong impression of the comparative risks of home and hospital births.

In 1980 the Social Services Committee of the House of Commons recommended that more women should be delivered in large units and home birth 'phased out further'.[3] It based this policy on a graph showing that more babies died at home than in hospital. Hidden in those statistics was the fact that unplanned out-of-hospital births accounted for the increase in deaths.[4]

66 If anything goes wrong in hospital, they say: "How lucky that you were in hospital!" They don't realise that it's because of what was done in hospital that things may have gone badly.

Women who have unplanned out-of-hospital births may be delivering long before the baby is ready for life, may be teenagers hiding a pregnancy and delivering somewhere—*anywhere*—where they hope their parents will not find out about the baby. They may be women delivering in a panic on the way to hospital, or they may be women who have had no antenatal care at all: the very poor, or women who are mentally confused, severely depressed, or addicted to drugs.

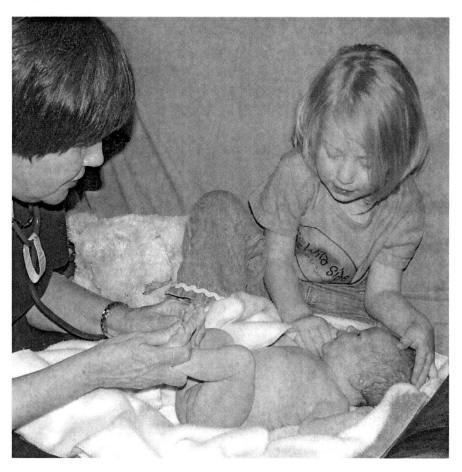

Home birth in different countries

All over the world caesarean section rates are on the increase. In Britain they have more than doubled in a generation, and over 100,000, caesareans are performed each year.[5] Although it might be expected that caesareans are replacing instrumental deliveries, this is not the case. Forceps and ventouse deliveries are also increasing. More and more women are having highly medicalised births.

At the same time women are expressing renewed interest in giving birth at home. In the Netherlands, where outcomes are very good, it is a straightforward matter to arrange this, and one third of all women have home births. It remains an exceptional country. Yet even where women give birth under the most centralised and authoritarian medical systems, such as in the former Soviet countries, women are wanting home births.

In Britain home births reached an all time low of less than 1% in the 1980s, but are now on the increase. 5,000 women a year have home births and the number is rising rapidly. In parts of the south west of England the proportion of home births is as high as 20% and many pregnant midwives themselves choose home births.

In the USA approximately 35,000 women a year give birth at home or in a free-standing birth centre. Many more would do so if there were the midwives to attend them, but midwives are few and far between. In Canada, following the legalisation of midwifery in some provinces, it is easier to get midwife care and midwives work both in hospitals and at home because they are allowed to attend home births.

In Western Australia professional caregivers working in hospitals are very disapproving of home births. As a result women who seek home birth, especially those who have had previous unhappy hospital experiences, are reluctant to be transferred even when there are clear signs that it would be safer for them and their babies to switch to hospital. When they are admitted women are separated from their own midwives, who must wait outside, and they often encounter punitive attitudes. This conflict between philosophies, fought out by those who should be giving service to childbearing women, wherever they are and whatever the circumstances, leads to confrontation and to delays in treatment, with home birth midwives and hospital doctors trying to prove their point.

The Australian situation is very different from that in countries where there is an established home birth service. Wherever women have to fight to get home birth they may do so even when they are potentially at high risk, believing that doctors are not telling them the truth and will not respect their wishes if they go into hospital. In Western Australia, for example, as many as 43% of multiparous women having home births in the 1980s had complications in previous births.[6] They were either ill-informed or were so scared of hospitals because of their previous experiences that they decided to take the risk. This is an indictment of a hospital system, not of the women who are abused by it.

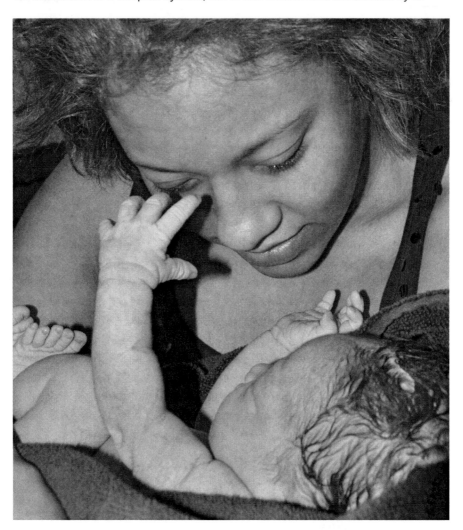

SAFETY

It may be useful to look at the Netherlands, where, still at the beginning of the 21st century, 38% of babies are born at home. Women having babies at home there may be cared for either by a midwife or a GP, and in hospital by midwives or doctors. If you look at baby deaths both in terms of where the birth took place and who attended the birth it emerges that care given by a midwife at home is safer than care from midwives in hospital, and home birth with a midwife is safest of all.[7]

A meta-analysis of the most reliable studies into planned home births in different countries, reveals that home birth is a valid alternative if you are not at special risk of difficulties in childbirth, and that women who give birth at home have fewer medical interventions.[8] The research covered 24,092 home births, matched with births to low risk women who were planning birth in hospital. Significantly fewer women who planned a home birth had their labours induced, received an episiotomy, or ended up with an operative vaginal delivery or caesarean section. They were less likely to have a bad perineal tear, and their babies were in better condition at birth. The conclusion was: "Home birth is an acceptable alternative to hospital confinement for selected pregnant women, and leads to reduced medical interventions."

It can be difficult to have a normal birth in hospital. Research into 6,000 planned home births in England and Wales revealed that women were one hundred times more likely to have labour induced if they planned a hospital birth, only 7% of women giving birth at home had their membranes artificially ruptured at or before 4cm dilation of the cervix, compared with 25% of those in hospital, and 8% received pethidine, compared with 30% in hospital.[9] Four times as many hospital mothers had a prolonged labour, and twice as many had an operative vaginal birth or caesarean section. Although few women actually haemorrhaged, twice as many women in hospital had heavy blood loss. At home women were more likely to have an intact perineum or, if they had a tear, only a first degree laceration, which is just a split in the skin, and does not damage muscle.

At home women were more likely to have an intact perineum or, if they had a tear, only a first degree laceration

The babies did better at home, too. Three times as many babies were recorded as having fetal distress in hospital. Twice as many had a low Apgar score (the examination that reveals if a newborn is lively) and more than twice as many needed oxygen.

For low risk mothers home birth is as safe, for both mother and baby, as hospital birth. In fact, it may be safer. So why was it, then, that in July 2010 the *American Journal of Obstetrics and Gynecology* published an article online by Wax, *et al.* that stated: "Less medical intervention during planned home birth is associated with a tripling of the neonatal mortality rates"?[10] And why was it that Professor Cathy Warwick, General Secretary of the Royal College of Midwives, responded immediately, saying that this was scaremongering, and criticising the *Lancet* for its editorial which said that women did not have the right to 'gamble' with their babies' health.[11] She was quoted in the *Guardian* as saying, "There is a danger that risk during childbirth is presented in a way which leads women to believe that hospital birth equals a safe birth, but it is not."[12] And why was it that a detailed critical appraisal soon followed from the Research Appraisal Trainer of the NCT (National Childbirth Trust), the Head of the Research and Information for the NCT, and the Professor of Perinatal Health at City University, London?[13]

The answer is simple: not only did the summary of births (which included 342,046 planned home births and 207,551 planned hospital births) confuse perinatal mortality and neonatal mortality, the methodology of the study overall was weak. Their finding that there was a two-fold higher rate for all planned home birth babies in what they called neonatal mortality, rising to a three-fold higher rate for those with congenital anomalies was unreliable because the research papers which Wax, *et al.* considered in their review were of widely varying quality and the different research papers did not consider the same data, so were not really comparable. Lumping them all together was simply not a valid research methodology... After all, some of the studies which were considered failed to distinguish stillbirths from babies who were born with congenital abnormalities. In one study deaths of twins and pre- and post-term babies were included in the home birth statistics but omitted from the hospital statistics. In another, deaths of babies in planned home births were stated but not in any birth signed by a medical professional. And the perinatal mortality rate was combined with the neonatal mortality rate, which will also have distorted the statistics. In any case, the study which contributed the most data to the neonatal mortality comparison used a methodology which is considered faulty.[14] This was because it took data from birth registers, which did not include a record of *planned* place of birth, meaning it's likely that unplanned home births were also included (which are widely recognised as being less safe.[15]) It was therefore completely unjustifiable to claim as they did in their abstract conclusion that "Less medical intervention during planned home birth is associated with a tripling of the neonatal mortality rate."[16] On the basis of the poor quality of their data, the authors should not have reached this conclusion. What they should have stated, if they had wanted to present their data in a straightforward way, was that—like previous researchers—they had found no difference in the safety of planned home birth and planned hospital birth for women without known risk factors when comparing perinatal mortality rates, which is the usual measure of safety.

> Like previous researchers, they had found no difference in the safety of planned home birth and planned hospital birth for women without known risk factors

It is, in fact, surprising that the editors of the *American Journal of Obstetrics and Gynecology* accepted the Wax paper for publication without major modifications.[17] If you doubt this, consider the comments made about the study by the chair of the American association CIMS (the Coalition for Improving Maternity Services), who commented that: "In our analysis of multiple studies from countries worldwide CIMS found that the authors of the study included confounding data, such as outdated and low-quality studies, low risk and high risk mothers, babies born preterm, babies unintentionally born at home, births attended by unqualified providers, and data from birth certificates, that researchers have found to be notoriously inaccurate."[18] Dr Michael Klein of the Child and Family Research Institute in Vancouver and Emeritus Professor of Family Practice and Paediatrics at the University of British Columbia, went as far as to assert that this study and the editorial which accompanied it constituted "an unabashed attempt to have poor science cover—unsuccessfully—a political agenda. I am very surprised that the (journal) would publish it."[19]

> It was called 'an unabashed attempt to have poor science cover—unsuccessfully—a political agenda

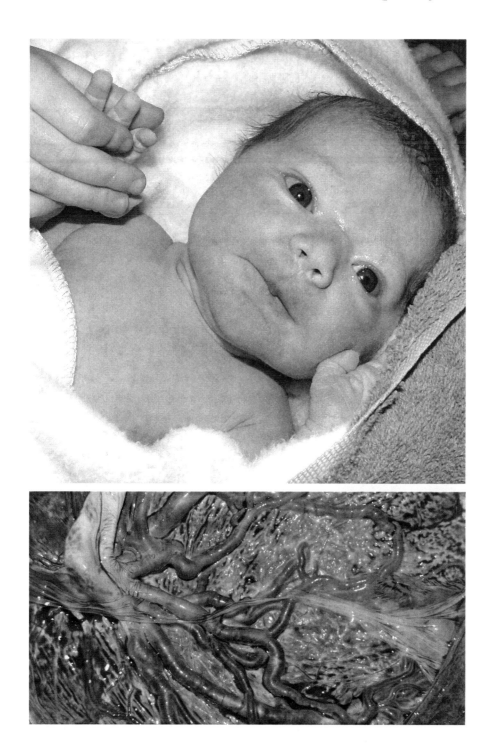

A CLOSER LOOK AT RISKS

Smoking

If you smoke, the single most important thing you can do to reduce risk to yourself and your baby is to stop smoking before you get pregnant or in the first half of the pregnancy, or at least to cut it down below 10 cigarettes a day.

> If you smoke, the single most important thing you can do to reduce risk to yourself and your baby is to stop smoking

Many midwives in the USA and Canada will not accept home birth clients who smoke during pregnancy, because of the associated risks.

> Nicotine constricts blood vessels so that the flow of blood through the placenta is slower, and this can lead to intra-uterine growth retardation (IUGR). Carbon monoxide and thiocynate in cigarette smoke also reduce the baby's growth.

Nicotine constricts blood vessels so that the flow of blood through the placenta is slower, and this can lead to intra-uterine growth retardation (IUGR). Carbon monoxide and thiocynate in cigarette smoke also reduce the baby's growth. Smokers are more at risk of miscarriage, of having pre-term babies, and of haemorrhage from the placenta. A woman who smokes and drinks alcohol takes even greater risks.

> Smokers are more at risk of miscarriage, of having pre-term babies, and of haemorrhage from the placenta

Alcohol

In North America fetal alcohol syndrome is the most usual teratogenic cause (that is, damage caused while the baby is in the uterus) of learning disabilities. This may occur when a woman drinks around eight glasses of wine or four pints of beer a day. You don't have to drink this much, however, to make it more likely that a baby will be born with low birth weight. There is some evidence that if you drink more than 10 glasses of wine a week the baby does not grow so well in the uterus.[20]

Your weight

If you are very underweight or overweight, this may affect your pregnancy and labour too. If you are very underweight, there is a chance that the baby will not be well nourished. If you are very fat, you are more likely to have raised blood pressure and to develop pregnancy diabetes, both of which will lead to your being advised not to give birth at home.[21]

Being fat means that you are also more likely to develop a urinary infection or to have a blood clot during pregnancy. But if you are healthy, there is no added risk to the baby; healthy overweight women give birth to healthy babies.[22] The customary practice of being weighed regularly in pregnancy, and all the worry that results, is worse than useless. However, if you want a home birth, it helps to be within a normal weight range. You and your caregivers are likely to feel happier about it. But, if you are overweight, never go on a crash diet during pregnancy. This is bad for both you and your baby. Ask for help from a dietician.

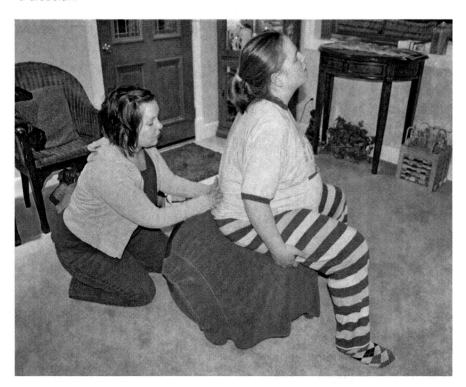

Your blood pressure

It is natural for blood pressure to rise a little at the very end of pregnancy.[23] But, if your blood pressure is up and at the same time protein (albumen) appears in your urine, you have pre–eclampsia and, unless it is very mild, you will usually be advised to have your baby in hospital, because the placenta may not be functioning well.

If your blood pressure is rising, look at ways in which you can cut down stress and take life easier. Pamper yourself and, if you possibly can, go to bed and ask other people to shop, cook, and clean. Listen to music, read, practise your relaxation, and get someone you love to massage you with a relaxing aromatherapy oil. If you already have children, this is very difficult to do unless there are other people close to you who can take over the children. You can always cuddle up with a toddler in bed, with picture books, television, and some new playthings, but two-year-olds are not the most restful little people to have around, and the therapy for your high blood pressure will have to be a compromise between care for yourself and the joys and responsibilities of mothering. Nevertheless, however you work it out, getting more rest gives you the best chance of being healthy at the end of the pregnancy, and still being able to have your baby at home. If this is your first baby, remember that once the baby is born you will never have the opportunity to lie around luxuriously like this again, so enjoy it!

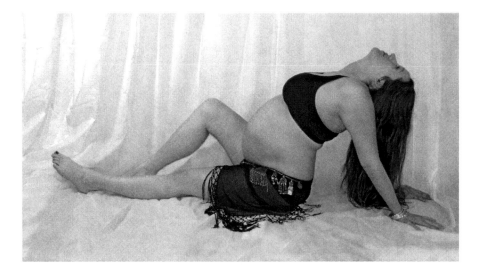

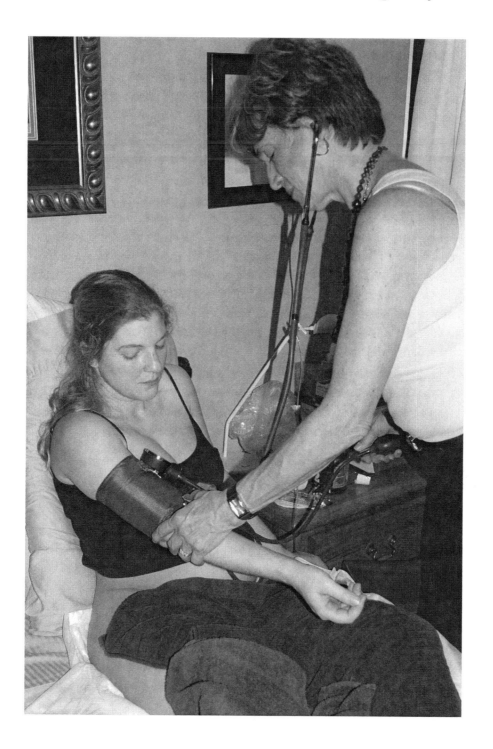

A breech baby

3 or 4 babies in every 100 are born bottom first.[24] Problems can arise because, although the baby's body may slip through easily, the birth of the head may be delayed, and this can result in oxygen deprivation.

3 or 4 babies in every 100 are born bottom first

In some countries caesarean sections are performed for most breech births, on the grounds that it is better to be safe than sorry. In Sweden, for example, nine out of ten breech babies are sections. Compare this with Norway, where only four or five are sections. If you live in a country where you know that if you have your baby in hospital you are more or less bound to have a caesarean, you may feel that a home or birth centre birth is an attractive alternative, as long as you can arrange for skilled and experienced care. On the other hand, you may find that your caregivers are very reluctant to take on the extra risk of a breech birth. To give you the best care at home, it is important that your midwife feels confident.

When interpreting statistics, bear in mind that many breech babies—more than 30%—are born like this because they are preterm (not yet 37 weeks). It is only as a baby becomes heavier that it tips head-down. If you go to term and have a breech baby, there is not the added risk that is associated with preterm babies.

When interpreting statistics, bear in mind that many breech babies—more than 30%—are born like this because they are preterm (not yet 37 weeks)

Babies who are breech in late pregnancy often somersault and are head-down by the time labour starts. About 14% are breech at 32 weeks.[25] and there is a 3 in 5 chance of them turning after that time, and still at 36 weeks a 1 in 4 chance,[26] although this is less likely if the baby's legs are extended, because legs splint the body, making it harder for the baby to roll over. Some babies even kick themselves round once labour has actually started, provided they have enough space.

External version in late pregnancy is successful in 60% of cases. It is an alternative to caesarean section. Be sure to ask for this if your baby is breech and you plan a home birth.

A previous preterm baby

If you have had a baby before who was born preterm, there is an increased possibility that this will happen again, but you still have an 83% chance of going to full term. Even if you have had two preterm births, there is still a 72% chance that this will not recur.[27]

A previous caesarean

If you have had a previous caesarean section, you will be advised by doctors to have your next baby and all other babies in hospital. Many obstetricians do repeat caesarean sections even when the same problems do not recur in another labour. (This is one reason why the caesarean section rate has rocketed in the UK, USA and elsewhere in the last 20 years.) Others allow a 'trial' of labour. This is really a trial of the scar, with everything ready for caesarean section in case it splits open. That means a hospital birth. However, rupture of the uterus occurs extremely rarely. In a series of 110,000 births following previous caesarean section there were 13 ruptures.[28]

Most of the papers in medical journals on which doctors base their policies warn against rupture following the old-fashioned 'classical' caesarean section, when the incision in the uterus is vertical. Nowadays most incisions are horizontal, in the lower segment of the uterus, just about at the level of the top of a bikini. The risks of rupture are much reduced when a horizontal, lower-segment incision has been made. With this kind of incision, even when the scar does not stand up to the strain of labour, it doesn't pop open, but one edge unpeels slightly—this is 'dehiscence'.

It is hard to know how to advise a woman who has had a caesarean section and who wants a home birth. There are additional risks in having a baby outside hospital, but there are also risks with unnecessary and harmful interventions that occur in many hospitals, and it may be that the previous caesarean section was the result of intervention.

> There are additional risks in having a baby outside hospital, but there are also risks with unnecessary and harmful interventions that occur in many hospitals, and it may be that the previous caesarean section was the result of intervention

MEDICAL CONDITIONS

Sometimes pregnant women are told by doctors that if they suffer from certain illnesses, such as diabetes, they must give birth in hospital. Doctors can make a strong case for diabetic mothers because, with all that sugar in the blood, babies often grow very large. In the past babies of diabetic mothers often had breathing problems. However, now that there is good insulin control during pregnancy, fewer than 2 in 100 have breathing problems.[29]

> With asthma there is no increased risk to the baby,
> and a good case for having a baby at home

Having said that, if you have an illness that gets worse when you are under stress, home may be the best place for you if you feel more secure and confident there. With asthma, for example, there is no increased risk to the baby, and a good case for having a baby at home.[30] With multiple sclerosis, home may be the ideal place too.[31]

> With multiple sclerosis, home may be the ideal place too

Rhesus negative mothers

Your blood is tested for the Rhesus factor in early pregnancy. If you are Rhesus negative and the baby's father is Rhesus positive, you have further tests later in pregnancy to find out whether you are developing antibodies to a Rhesus positive baby. This is extremely unlikely to happen if it is your first baby and if you have not had a previous miscarriage, but the risk increases if anything is done that causes bleeding in pregnancy, such as chorionic villus sampling, amniocentesis, and fetoscopy.

Interventions during labour and at delivery can also cause leaking of the baby's blood into your own and result in sensitisation in the next pregnancy. These include fixing a scalp clip to the baby's head to monitor the heart rate, forceps delivery or caesarean section, accidental tearing of the cord if it is pulled in an attempt to deliver the placenta, and manual removal of the placenta. So childbirth without unnecessary intervention is the safest course of action, which may mean that birth at home or in a birth centre is best.

Fewer than 1 baby in 1,000 dies today from problems associated with Rhesus incompatibility. If you do not develop antibodies during pregnancy, your baby and you are not at increased risk. You should be able to choose the place where you would like to have your baby.

The discovery of gamma-globulin in the 1960s, and its regular use now when a Rhesus negative woman is likely to be bearing a Rhesus positive baby, has saved many lives. The woman has injections of anti-D immunoglobulin during pregnancy, at the birth, or within five days of the birth of a Rhesus positive baby to avoid sensitisation in the next pregnancy, and will be screened regularly during later pregnancies.

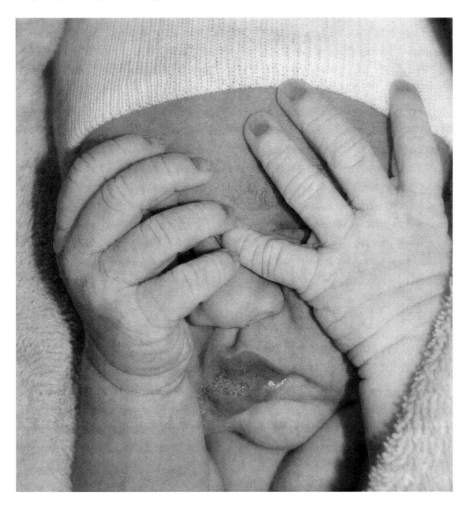

MYTHS ABOUT HOME BIRTH

"Older mothers shouldn't have home births"

If you are having your first baby over the age of 35, or with some doctors even over 30, you are considered an 'elderly primigravida', at greater risk of what obstetricians sometimes call 'poor obstetric performance'. Some even describe older mothers as 'obstetrically senescent' or 'geriatric'.[32]

Nowadays women having their first baby in their 30s have not necessarily had a long history of fertility problems—something associated with increased risk—but have delayed motherhood because of their careers or until they felt ready to have a child. Their education and socio-economic conditions mean that they are in a low risk group compared with, say, teenagers who become pregnant accidentally or because they want someone to love. The perinatal mortality rate for these older mothers is no higher than that for younger mothers.[33]

What is different is the amount of obstetric intervention that older mothers receive in hospital. In one London hospital women over 35 were more than twice as likely to have labour augmented with oxytocin (53% compared with 20% of under-35s), more likely to have an episiotomy (74% compared with 38%), more likely to be delivered by forceps (35% compared with 25%) and more likely to have a caesarean section (28% compared with 13%).[34] The high caesarean rate may occur because more older mothers receive continuous electronic monitoring, and anxiety on the part of obstetricians may contribute to the aggressive management of labour. One way of avoiding this, a valid option if you have a healthy pregnancy, is to have your baby in a birth centre or at home.

"A long labour at home is dangerous"

It is tiring when the cervix dilates slowly but, unless other problems develop, it is not dangerous. Labours that last more than 48 hours in hospital often lead to forceps delivery, vacuum extraction or caesarean section, which may themselves introduce risk. At home you can have a more relaxed attitude to time. There is no relation between long labour (over 24 hours) and learning disabilities in babies.[35]

Cephalo-pelvic disproportion (CPD), where the baby's head is too big to pass through the mother's pelvis is often misdiagnosed simply because labour is long. When a woman is in labour at home and it becomes obvious that the baby is having difficulty passing through her pelvis it is sensible to transfer to hospital. This is not a sudden emergency. It is a decision made following discussion when it is clear that no progress is being made.

A general practitioner having her first baby:

66 Midwives carry oxygen to give a baby if necessary, but the doctors I saw didn't realise that. I want a home birth because I am anxious to avoid my delivery becoming as medicalised as those I witnessed during my training.

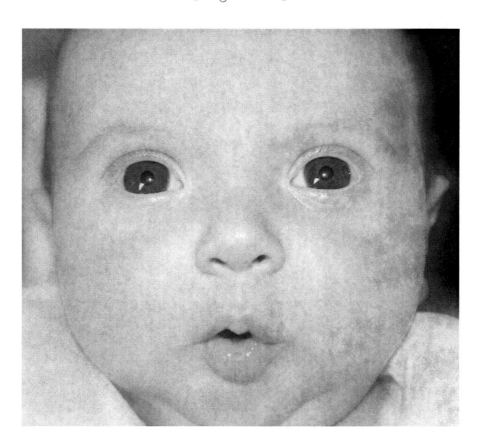

"If the baby has breathing problems nothing can be done"

Babies are most likely to have breathing difficulties when their mothers have had pain-killing drugs in labour, including pethidine, sedatives, tranquillizers, and epidural anaesthesia. A woman having a baby at home often has no drugs at all or, if she chooses to have them, only a very small dose. Simple ways of resuscitating a baby—clearing the airways, giving oxygen and massage—can be used at home.

"Women have to be in hospital in case they haemorrhage"

Postpartum haemorrhage (heavy bleeding) is most likely to occur when there has been obstetric intervention in birth or attempts have been made to pull the placenta out before it has completely separated from the uterine wall. If there is bleeding, syntometrine (artificial oxytocin) can be given by injection to make the uterus contract firmly, and it is simple to do this at home.

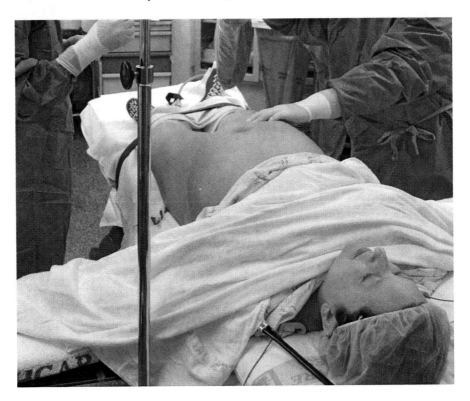

THE BABY'S SAFETY

Whenever a woman decides to have a home birth, there are people who suggest that either the baby might die from neglect because it is not born in a hospital setting, or that it might be mentally damaged from lack of oxygen. The perinatal mortality rate for planned home births is very low indeed—3 to 4 per 1,000 compared with 8 per 1,000 births overall.

The perinatal mortality rate for planned home births is very low indeed: 3 to 4 per 1,000 compared with 8 per 1,000 overall

Moreover, two of these three or four deaths are unavoidable wherever the baby is born, because the baby is extremely preterm or suffers a congenital abnormality that is incompatible with life. All that birth in a high-tech hospital might do is delay death by a few days or weeks.

92% of all learning disabilities in babies occur *before* labour, either as the result of congenital malformation (around 63%) or events and processes that occurred during pregnancy, such as intra-uterine growth retardation (8%), infections such as rubella (6%), or accidents such as lead poisoning. The damage occurred long before labour started.[32]

66 *Working in an intensive care unit, I see many babies being kept alive who I think should have been allowed to die in peace. That's one reason why I've decided on a home birth.*

In a hospital with an intensive care unit a baby with severe learning disabilities is taken immediately to have all the life-saving procedures that are available. Being in hospital may make the difference between death and survival with a major handicap. Some women choose home birth because they would not want vigorous and extraordinary methods to be used to save the life of a damaged baby. Others choose hospital because they want the baby to have every chance of life, however severe its disabilities.

Some women choose hospital because they want the baby to have every chance of life, however severe its disabilities

OPTIMISING CONDITIONS

It is an enormous responsibility to bring a baby into the world and it starts long before the baby is in your arms. There are doctors who accuse women having a home birth of 'child abuse', and who would even like to prosecute them. They see it as a choice only a selfish woman would make and see themselves as the saviours of babies, rescuing them from their egotistical, hysterical mothers. Yet your informed decision to give birth at home or in a birth centre can be one way to accept deep personal responsibility for your baby.

Accept deep personal responsibility for your baby

If you want to have your baby at home, it makes sense to:

♥ Find a good midwife. She should be skilled, confident, and relaxed in working in an out-of-hospital setting.

♥ Get all the information you can about how to help yourself. Learn the art of meeting contractions with relaxation, breathing and focused concentration, and find out how a variety of positions and movements can assist descent and rotation of the baby. Approach birth free from fear, self-assured and positive.

♥ Have more than one birth attendant. Your caregivers need to work well together: a midwife needs her own support. Immediately after the birth you and the baby may need attention at the same time.

♥ Ensure that you have access to a telephone. It is useful to have a car if you can, just in case it is needed.

♥ The midwife should have simple equipment such as a Pinard stethoscope or, better still, a Sonicaid; drugs to make the uterus contract after the baby is born if you bleed a good deal; the skills to help you handle pain, perhaps with hot compresses, a bath, shower or birthing pool; and she should carry oxygen in case it is needed.

♥ Make certain that your home is reasonably clean, comfortable, and convenient for giving birth, with hot and cold water, some form of heating in cold weather and a way to cool the air in hot weather.

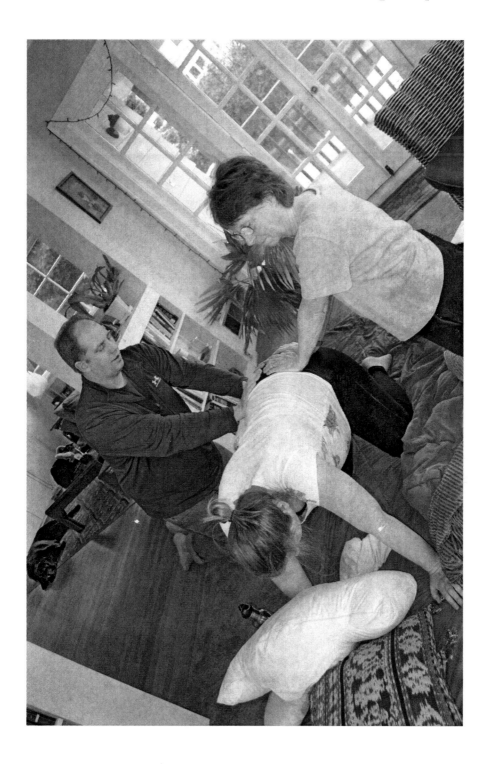

Making arrangements

Depending on where you live, you may have the choice between giving birth in a birth centre run by midwives, linked with or completely separate from a hospital, a small GP unit, or at home. It is worth exploring your options.

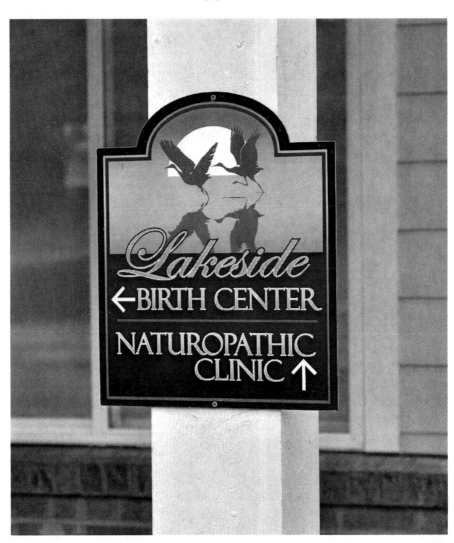

THE BIRTH CENTRE: HOME FROM HOME?

A birth centre, at least ideally, provides exclusively low-technology care, there is a homely atmosphere, and you return home a matter of hours after giving birth. In the United States, where the first birth centre was established in New York in 1975, birth centres have mushroomed. The same applies to the UK. (To find where there are birth centres near you, simply go to www.birthchoiceuk.com and enter your postcode. Birth centres are 'Midwife or GP led units' or 'Midwife or GP led unit, co-located with a consultant unit.' Alternatively, locate a birth centre at the website www.babycentre.co.uk—by clicking on 'Pregnancy', 'Labour & birth', 'Planning birth', 'Birth centres' and 'How can I find out more about birth centres?') Caregivers in birth centres are for the most part nurse direct-entry midwives or nurses working with an obstetrician, although in some centres there are direct-entry midwives with no nursing background.

A birth centre may be free-standing, in hospital grounds, or inside a hospital building. The important thing about it is that it should have a distinct atmosphere of its own and its special staff. The policy of the Family Health Program Birth Center in Salt Lake City, in the USA, for example, is "to provide safe maternity care to low risk families, in a home-like, out-of-hospital setting," and achieve "parental satisfaction through a highly educational, personalised form of care, which encourages intra-family contact and participation in the management... of childbearing. Childbirth is a peak life experience and is viewed as a healthy process. Confidence in the physiologic function of the body to cope with childbirth is promoted in all aspects of care." Health care providers are educators and resource people to enable women to take responsibility for their own health.

> As much obstetric intervention is likely to take place in beautifully decorated rooms (with paintings on the walls, flowered wallpaper, hanging plants and rocking chairs) as in the more clinical-looking rooms along the corridor

Some hospitals have introduced birth rooms with paintings on the walls, flowered wallpaper, hanging plants and rocking chairs, but there is no special philosophy of care that arises from a holistic approach to childbirth, and as much obstetric intervention is likely to take place in these rooms as in the more clinical-looking rooms along the corridor.

How is a birth centre different from a hospital?

In a birth centre worthy of the name:

- ♥ There is no induction.

- ♥ There is no augmentation of labour with oxytocin.

- ♥ There is no electronic fetal monitoring except for Doppler ultrasound—when a Sonicaid is used.

- ♥ There are no epidurals.

- ♥ There are very few episiotomies.

- ♥ There are no operative deliveries (forceps or ventouse, or caesareans).

In many birth centres the only types of equipment are oxygen tanks and catheters for clearing a baby's airways when they are blocked, and local anaesthesia to suture tears in the perineum.

In the Garden of Life Birth Center in Dearborn, Michigan in the USA, where the focus is on cultural sensitivity to the needs of the Muslim, Italian, Hispanic, Polish and Anglo parents using the centre, the sole machinery is a coffee-maker. Staff wear ordinary clothing, not uniforms. Women can move around in labour and adopt any position they like for birth. Childbirth education is an integral part of the programme, and other members of the family can be present at the birth. The bed is king-sized, low, and comfortable, so that mother, father, and new baby can cuddle together.

❝ I saw my baby's head crowning and she was placed on my tummy. No tubes were forced down her throat. She was born amid laughter and joy, shared by all. Our second child is almost due and will be born in the same peaceful, gentle atmosphere of Boothville.

❝ I enjoyed being looked after as a Special Mum, as everyone was treated there, and I treasure the warmth and fun that was shared with those midwives and doctors.

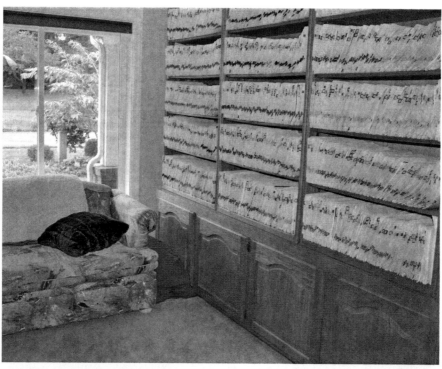

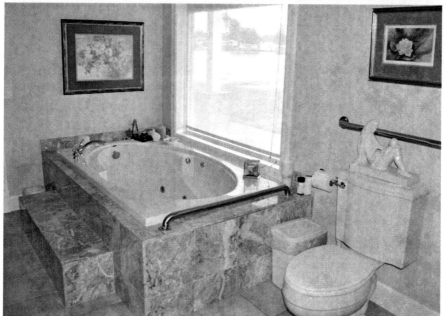

Can anyone use a birth centre?

Birth centres tend to have very strict rules as to who may use them. Some, such as the New York Maternity Childbearing Center, screened out half of the women who applied. (Unfortunately, that particular centre has since closed down.) Women may be screened out partly because of legal or insurance restrictions, and partly because many birth centres are administered or funded by a health authority or hospital. Women who are screened out may include:

♥ women expecting twins

♥ women with pre-eclampsia

♥ women with diabetes

♥ women who develop problems during pregnancy—suspected fetal growth retardation, for instance

Midwives and nurses working independently in birth centres and small clinics, even in countries where midwifery is already a strong profession, as in Sweden, find a satisfying new role and exciting relationship with the families they are helping. In a birth centre in Stockholm, for example, it is a midwife, not a doctor, who makes the decision as to whether labour is deviating from the norm and who then refers a woman to obstetric care in the same building. In that birth centre such a referral happens with 1 woman in 10 during pregnancy. In the early days a further 30% of women were moved during labour, often for oxytocin stimulation of the uterus because their waters had broken and there were no contractions, or labour was slow, but as midwives became more confident this very high percentage of transfers was halved in the first six months the birth centre was open. In most American birth centres between 7% and 16% of women are switched to obstetric care because they require drugs for pain relief, have slow labours, or there is failure to progress. You will need to bear this in mind if you decide you would like to give birth in a birth centre, even though transfer is just a small possibility.

At the Edgware Birth Centre near London, where 387 gave birth over a two-year period, only six women had an episiotomy. That is a rate of 1.5% compared with a rate of 11.0% for women who had normal births in local hospitals. Half of the birth centre mothers gave birth in a pool.[1]

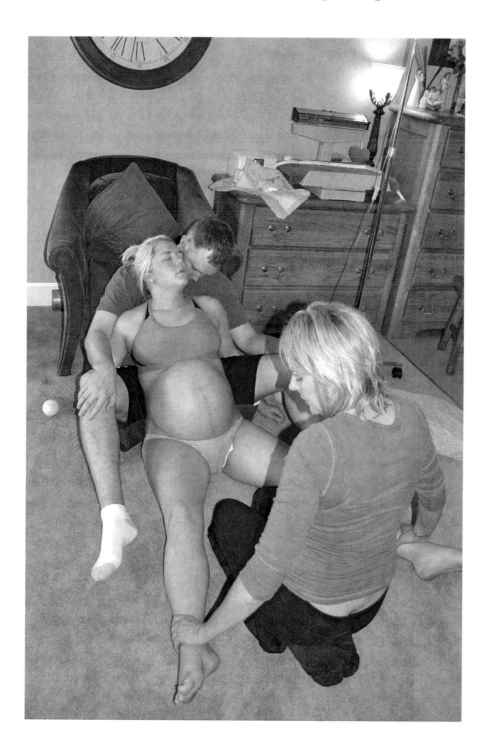

Why choose a birth centre?

In Britain, birth centres—both within the National Health Service and privately run, but often selling their service to NHS trusts—are now part of a rapidly developing movement aimed at woman-centred care. They fill the gap that resulted from the closing down of many small maternity units run by midwives and GPs and the difficulty that women experience in getting home births. All over the country these small birth units have been closed on the grounds that they are uneconomical and that it is safer for all births to be concentrated in large regional hospitals. The evidence for the increased safety for low risk mothers in large hospitals is unconvincing, and these cottage-type birth units were held in great affection in their communities, but they were shut down all the same. Their destruction has left a huge gap. Women may have to travel great distances to hospital, and they are less likely to be able to get to know the midwives who attend them in childbirth. The intimacy and friendliness of care is often lost in the large institutions which replaced them.

> 66 It is a relaxed, caring, warm and friendly environment where you count as a person and not a number on a conveyor belt.

Now birth centres are eagerly sought by women who dislike the impersonality of hospital. They want to have people around them whom they know; they want to retain control over what happens to them; and they want to labour without drugs or interventions. The Edgware Birth Centre, in London, for example, which was within the NHS, was booked solid and could not keep up with demand. (Unfortunately, it has since closed down.)

> Women who choose to give birth in a birth centre
> want to have people around them who they know
> and they want to retain control over what happens to them

It is not just pregnant women who may prefer birth in a small midwife-run centre. Midwives, lacking job satisfaction in large hierarchical, bureaucratic systems in which their skills are downgraded, look to these birth centres as places where they can give the kind of care which was the reason why they entered the profession. For some midwives, birth centres hold the promise of a rebirth of midwifery.

In a good birth centre you can expect architecture on a human scale and attractive interior design

In a good birth centre you can expect architecture on a human scale and attractive interior design, with such things as comfortable furniture, photographs of the midwives with their names on the noticeboard, and many photographs of mothers with their new babies, pictures, sculptures, mobiles, and other representations of birth. Rooms are often carpeted, lighting can be dimmed, there are curtains at the windows, beanbags and relaxation chairs, maybe a patchwork quilt, and a wooden crib or muslin-hung cot. You have your own bathroom with a large bathtub, perhaps a jacuzzi, and a powerful shower for back massage. There may be a birthing pool in which you can labour and give birth if you wish. The atmosphere is relaxing and non-clinical, offering a space in which you and your partner can be private, locking the door when you want to. No shiny instruments are in evidence, although there may be some tucked behind the curtain. You can bring in things you would like to have around you and wear your own clothes, not institutional garb.

You can bring in things you would like to have around you

The kitchen is often located centrally in the building and is a gathering place for expectant parents, midwives, and new parents as they talk over cups of tea. In the Stockholm Birth Centre parents have their own fridge and make meals when they want them. No one serves up meals at set times. The father or mother, or perhaps a grandparent, makes a snack whenever they wish. In a very different birth centre in El Paso, Texas, the kitchen is also the heart of the centre but, in contrast to the style of the modern white-wood Swedish kitchen with its bundles of dried rosebuds, this is a Mexican kitchen, familiar and comforting for the mothers who walk across the border in labour to give birth in the United States, hoping that in this way their babies may become American citizens. Instead of Swedish cheese and shortbread cookies, they sniff the odours of Mexican dishes based on black beans and peppers.

Antenatal care is given by midwives, who may talk through emotional aspects of the birth experience with you for as long as two hours. They're unlikely to limit care simply to the administration of tests. In fact, in some birth centres you are shown how to test your urine and check your own blood pressure at home.

Choosing a good birth centre

Unfortunately, there are many phoney birth centres. As health care entrepreneurs and hospital administrators have caught on to the birth centre as a major marketing opportunity—a venture that could make their hospital more competitive with others—the original concept has been diluted.

Those who own a birth centre—business people, doctors, a health authority, hospital, or whatever—control how it is run and everything that happens in it. If a birth centre is not run by the midwives who work in it, be particularly careful about examining the pros and cons of that particular centre.

> Just because a maternity unit is called a birth centre,
> do not assume that care is woman-centred

Just because a maternity unit is called a birth centre, do not assume that care is woman-centred. For example, in US birth centres, 15% of women have intravenous infusions. Also, the typical Californian centre is physician-owned in a commercial building, with a couple of birth rooms, and births are attended by obstetricians. Californian physician-owned insurance companies will not usually provide malpractice cover for birth centres unless they are on hospital grounds, and only obstetricians can do deliveries. Malpractice insurance is too high for most family practitioners to risk working in a birth centre, and nurse-midwives have great difficulty in obtaining insurance cover to work there unless they are supervised by an obstetrician.

66 It's run by a cosmetic surgeon, with an obstetrician on call. He has an office downstairs where he does the cosmetic surgery.

In the United States non-profit institutions staffed by nurse-midwives or registered midwives with back-up from a sympathetic obstetrician are giving way to hundreds of profit centres, and, as in Australia, hospitals offer birth rooms as a cosmetic exercise to attract more customers. Yet the non-profit birth centres that can still be found often provide most value for money: offering more childbirth education, more antenatal care, more classes for siblings, and more home visits after the birth.

Along with the increase in physician-operated centres, some American obstetricians have equipped their offices to do out-of-hospital births, both in response to consumer demand and to make a fast buck. Procedures used may include paracervical blocks (pain-killing injections around the cervix), electronic fetal monitoring, ultrasound, induction and augmentation of labour, vacuum extraction, forceps, and even, in at least one birth centre, caesarean section.

❝ I was told that every first-time mother had Demerol (pethidine). It wasn't a question of whether she thought she needed it.

As obstetricians take over the birth centre movement, they also transfer their concept of birth as a medical event, and with it there is increasing dependence on technology.

❝ There is a time-limit on labour, and then they shove you in a hospital. This hospital has a 30% caesarean rate.

Questions to ask

When enquiring about a particular birth centre, you may want to ask these questions:

♥ What is your transfer rate during pregnancy? (This will enable you to estimate what your chances are of actually having your baby in the birth centre.)

♥ What is your transfer rate during labour? (A rate of between 7% and 12% is reasonable.)

♥ Do you ever induce labour?

♥ Is electronic fetal monitoring used? (Doppler ultrasound for intermittent monitoring is acceptable, in the form of a hand-held Sonicaid. Scalp clips and abdominal belts are not.)

♥ Is intravenous glucose given?

♥ Are pain-relieving drugs used?

♥ Do you offer epidural anaesthesia?

♥ Is labour ever augmented?

♥ Is there a time limit on the second stage?

♥ What percentage of women have episiotomies? (It should be less than 10%.)

♥ Do you ever do forceps delivery or vacuum extraction?

The answers to these questions may make you want to ask more. If any procedures are used, it will help to know if they are employed more or less routinely or rarely, so you may wish to ask for percentages of different interventions in the previous year. Other questions concern your freedom to do whatever you feel like doing at the time:

♥ Can I walk around during labour?

♥ Can I give birth on the floor if I wish?

♥ Do women ever give birth standing up?

♥ How do you help a woman with backache labour?

♥ Can I get in the bath or shower during labour?

♥ What do you do when dilation is slow?

♥ Is it possible for my other children to be present?

♥ May I eat and drink during labour if I want to?

♥ Will there be a midwife or maternity nurse with me all the time through the late first stage?

♥ Can I use a birthing pool?

Again, although the answers will give you an idea of the quality of care, your spontaneous feelings are also a good guide. Your intuitive reactions about whether this is the place in which you would like to give birth are important. You need to feel relaxed, confident, secure, and among friends.

Birth centres have proved safe, and in many of them few invasive, uncomfortable, restrictive procedures are used during birth. In the United States a national study of 11,814 women admitted to 84 free–standing birth centres revealed that the perinatal mortality rate was as low as 1.3 per 1,000 births compared with 8.0 per 1,000 for all hospital births.[2]

In New York outcomes for low risk mothers booked at the Maternity Center's Childbearing Center were compared with those for low risk mothers at a large teaching hospital, Mount Sinai. Women in hospital were more likely to have labour induced, and augmentation of labour occurred six times as frequently. Amniotomy more than two hours before the birth was more common; electronic fetal monitoring was used five times as often; four times as many women laboured with intravenous drips set up; more than double the number had drugs for pain relief; and there were eleven times as many epidurals. Women in the birth centre had noticeably longer second stages: over 80% had second stages lasting more than two hours, compared with fewer than 19% in the hospital. The incidence of thick meconium staining was three times greater for women in the hospital. (When some of the contents of the baby's bowel appear like this during labour, it can be a sign that the baby is over-stressed.) Women in the birth centre were four times as likely to have an intact perineum—that is, no tear and no episiotomy. Judging by live, healthy babies, birth was just as safe in the Childbearing Center as at this prestigious hospital, but with far less intervention and in a pleasanter environment.

In hospitals, even those advocating 'family-centred' care, intervention rates are much higher. Research in Australian hospitals reveals that those with flexible policies aiming for sensitivity to parents' wishes still have high rates of induction of labour, oxytocin use, and operative deliveries.[3]

❝ Everything was warm, friendly, and fuss-free. My husband was tired after a long flight, and as I was walking about and leaning on Sue, my midwife, when I had a contraction, and was in and out of the bath, she tucked him up in the bed for a snooze whilst we got on with it. Then, when contractions were coming every two minutes, she woke him up with a cup of tea so that he didn't miss anything. She showed him how to rub my back and we made a great team!

In birth centres or birth rooms that are an integral part of a hospital the orientation towards treating patients as high risk and using all techniques available spills over to low risk women across the corridor. This takes place even though the benefits are marginal or non-existent and the interventions are sometimes harmful. In a Canadian hospital, for example, as many as 63% of first-time mothers and 19% of those who had already had babies were transferred from the birth room to the conventional hospital setting.[4] Clearly, if you are choosing a birth centre linked to a hospital, it is essential that it has its own staff and that they are confident and skilled enough to give continuing, low-technology care.

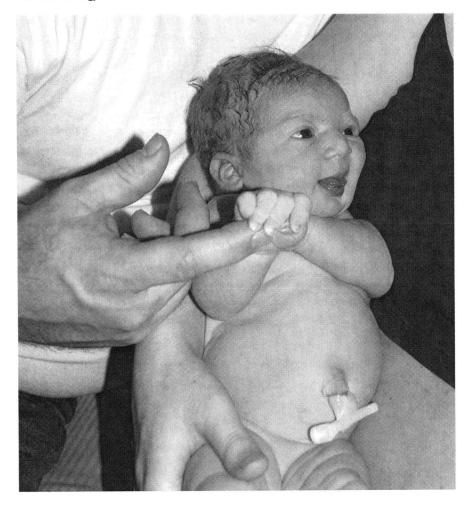

Birth centre Q&A:

Q: Can anyone use a birth centre?

A: Birth centres are for low risk women. If you are expecting twins, have pre-eclampsia or diabetes, or develop pregnancy problems, you may have to negotiate to give birth there.

Q: Are all birth centres run along the same lines?

A: No. A set of rooms in a hospital decorated to look attractive, but that is not run by midwives, is a birth centre in name only.

Q: Are birth centres safe?

A: Birth centres have proved themselves safe and in most of them, few invasive, uncomfortable or restrictive procedures are used. In the United States a study of 11,814 women admitted to 84 free-standing birth centres revealed that the perinatal mortality rate was as low as 1.3 per 1,000 births compared with 8 per 1,000 for all hospital births.[2]

Q: What sort of atmosphere can I expect?

A: The atmosphere is relaxing and non-clinical, and there is little or no intervention. You have a private room with soft lighting, comfortable furniture and equipment that enables you to be upright and to move around during labour. You can bring things you would like to have and wear your own clothes.

Q: What is antenatal care like?

A: Antenatal care is from midwives who give one-to-one care, discuss with you the emotional aspects of the birth experience, and do not limit care to doing tests and recording results. In some birth centres you are also shown how to check your own urine and blood pressure at home.

Q: And postnatal care?

A: Your baby is able to stay with you round the clock, and your partner too. You are given strong support for breastfeeding. You and your partner can be private—even lock the door—and other children and family members are welcomed.

MIDWIFERY-LED UNITS — SMALL IS BEAUTIFUL?

Midwifery-led units (sometimes called general practitioner units), are often housed within a larger hospital and are sometimes isolated. They exist in the UK and other European countries, and in Australia and New Zealand and grew out of community cottage hospitals.

These small units are often homely and welcoming. Women like them because they already know the midwives and/or doctor, mothers and babies are kept together after birth as a matter of course, and they are near home. It is usually not possible to have an epidural or caesarean section in a small unit like this, and a baby who needs special care must be moved to where there are intensive care facilities. Some midwifery-led units are quite old-fashioned, but have kept the best of the old and incorporated active childbirth and gentle birth into their practice. Many have also only recently been set up. The emphasis is usually on as little intervention as possible during birth and on a close, supportive relationship between the midwife and her client.

Midwifery-led units (or GP units) have a good safety record, whether they are isolated or annexed to a larger hospital. In New Zealand, for example, babies of normal birth weight are more likely to die in large, high-tech hospitals than in small maternity units.[5]

Choosing a midwifery-led unit or GP unit

If you are considering a midwifery-led unit, or a GP unit, visit it first and ask the same questions that you might ask of a birth centre (see pages 93-94), including the rate of transfer. You will probably have a one-to-one relationship with the midwife because she is attached to your GP's practice, so you will be able to ask her how she avoids episiotomies, what she recommends if a woman has a slow, backache labour, how she feels about waterbirth, and so on. With a good midwife this type of dialogue is a vital part of your relationship with her. Midwives create the flavour of a unit. In some areas they are attached to the unit rather than to a hospital or a GP practice, so you may not meet them unless you go to the unit. Protocols for units are usually strict. You won't find high-tech gadgets sneaked in or interventionist obstetric techniques employed, although you may find that an amniotomy is done (the bag of waters gets broken). It is likely that you will find midwives who are keen for you to walk about during labour or soak in a bath, and who know how to help you have a physiological rather than a managed birth.

You may have the option of a small maternity unit that is staffed and run by midwives. They are very similar to those units that are separate from large hospitals and the atmosphere is warm, friendly and relaxed. There is usually a good system of obstetric back-up combined with personal care from midwives whom you get to know before the birth.

66 The doctor tried to persuade me to go into the GP unit. He said it was 'homely' and I could do just what I wanted there. But there's a vast difference between someone else's place being 'homely' and my own home.

Unfortunately, as we have seen, in most industrialised countries in Europe, North America and Australia governments are closing down small hospitals and outlying midwifery-led units or GP units—in spite of a great deal of protest from consumers—on the grounds of safety, 'rationalisation', and economics. They are concentrating care in large regional centres with high-tech facilities in great gleaming edifices of steel and glass. With regionalisation of care, women have to travel long distances when they go to antenatal appointments and also when they go into hospital early on in labour. Moreover, care in these hospitals is focused on pathology and it tends to be less flexible and more impersonal than in small hospitals. There is often severe overcrowding in antenatal clinics, with long waiting times, and women are herded through them like cattle. Authoritarian attitudes set administrative convenience before the needs of the women for whom the service is supposed to exist.[6]

Many midwifery-led GP units have, at least potentially, the qualities of a good birth centre (and some midwifery-led units are even called 'birth centres'), and they offer a similar relaxed kind of care. Without either midwifery-led units (MLUs) or GP units, women are forced into standard hospital care, with its high intervention rates, unless they decide on a home birth. Actually, if you are considered sufficiently low risk to be allowed to give birth in any of these small maternity units, you might also think about the option of a home birth. Birth centres, MLUs and GP units are for women who are expected to have normal births, and if it is a sensible choice to give birth in a unit like this, it is equally safe, or even safer, to give birth at home.

If it is sensible to give birth in a midwifery-led unit or GP unit, it's equally safe, or safer to give birth at home

One of the strongest arguments against having your baby anywhere else is that once a woman is in an institution interventions can take place that no midwife or doctor would be likely to attempt at home. Even in small maternity units there is a risk that a physiological labour may be turned into a managed labour just because you are in a place where medical hardware is available, and where professionals make the decisions.

One of the strongest arguments against having your baby anywhere apart from at home is that once a woman is in an institution interventions can take place

Midwifery-led unit and GP unit Q&A:

Q: What are midwifery-led units (MLUs) and GP units?

A: Free-standing midwifery-led units and general practitioner units, sometimes isolated, such as exist in the UK and other European countries, and in Australia and New Zealand, grew out of cottage hospitals serving the community. They are all really midwifery units. They cater for low risk women only.

Q: Will I be able to have an active birth in an MLU or GP unit?

A: Some of these small hospitals are quite old-fashioned, but many have kept the best of the old and incorporated active childbirth and gentle birth into their practice.

Q: Will my GP or a consultant look after me?

A: No. Although beds in GP units are called 'GP beds', most care is by midwives. The GP may not even turn up for the birth.

Q: Who can use a midwifery-led or GP unit?

A: Women who are expected to have normal births. The transfer rate to hospital because of unexpected complications is anything from 7%-30%. It's worth asking what the transfer rate is.

GP units are midwifery units—and are only for low risk women

Points to consider

- ♥ Is there a midwifery-led unit or GP unit sufficiently close to my home?

- ♥ If I need to be transferred to hospital during labour how far will I have to travel, and what kind of care can I expect from that hospital?

- ♥ Will I be able to choose the type of birth I want for myself and my baby and will I be free to make my own decisions?

- ♥ Will I have a chance to get to know my carers during pregnancy and discuss my choices for the birth before I go into labour?

Find out whether or not you'll be able to make your own decisions about the kind of care you receive and whether or not you'll get to know your caregivers in advance

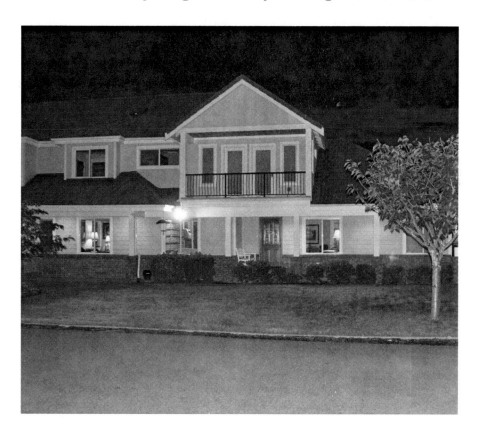

AT HOME

The essential difference between giving birth at home and giving birth in even the most peaceful, pleasant birth room in an institution is the knowledge that home is your space, the place that you control, and where other people come as guests.

❝ I went to my doctor expecting opposition and he said, "What a good idea!"

❝ There is a genuine friendship with a doctor who shares your conviction that home is the best place, and who supports you.

If you have decided that you will feel more secure, more confident, and more relaxed giving birth at home, the first step is to find out what is available in your area. In Britain you do not require a doctor's consent to have a home birth. You can make arrangements directly with a midwife. But unless you live in a place where there are keen homebirth midwives, arranging a home birth may not be easy. You have to ask yourself:

♥ Can I summon up the stamina, courage, and persistence to overcome obstacles that are likely to be put in my way?

♥ Where can I obtain the emotional support and practical help from other people that I shall need?

♥ Can I be assertive enough to state what I want, avoiding both aggression and submission?

♥ Can I be assertive enough to negotiate the care that I believe is right for me and my baby?

❝ "You do realise," he said, "that home birth is child abuse? We've got a perfectly good hospital here offering family-centred care."

The essential difference between giving birth at home and giving birth in an institution is the knowledge that home is your space

The first challenge may be to obtain information about who can help if your doctor refuses a home birth. One of the organisations listed in the Useful contacts (at the back of this book) will be able to put you in touch with a group in your area. Working your way past other people's non-comprehension, criticism, and their sometimes punitive responses, may be rather like finding your way through a baffling maze. But it can also be exciting!

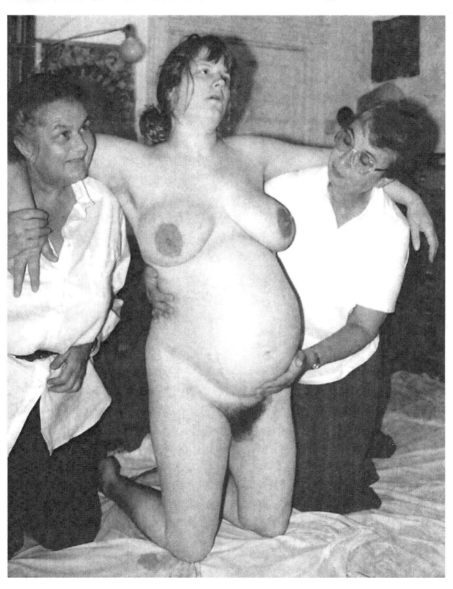

Talking to your doctor

Do not attempt to broach the subject when you are flat on your back with your legs in the air. Make certain that you are sitting face-to-face with the doctor. Settle back comfortably in the chair, avoid fiddling nervously with your clothes, hands or bag, and look the doctor straight in the eye.

> 66 The doctor told me he wouldn't do a home birth because "my place on the committee would be in jeopardy," and said, "If you have a home delivery, everyone'll want one!"

> 66 What is important is the attitude you have to authority. To have a home birth, you have to be willing to question and to challenge authority.

Rehearse what you are going to say beforehand with someone sympathetic. It helps to have someone who knows what doctors may say in these situations. Remember that most doctors are frightened of home births because they have no experience of them. You don't have to go into lengthy explanations or make a speech, to defend or excuse yourself, to quote statistics, or to placate the doctor. Refuse to be drawn into arguments. All you need do is say clearly and firmly that you want a home birth, and, if you wish, give a simple explanation of why. You may have to repeat it over and over again, a technique sometimes known as 'the cracked record'. Afterwards, discuss with someone close to you how you each felt at different stages of the conversation, and at the end of it.

If you find this difficult, you can rehearse the interview by yourself, sitting in front of a mirror. Talk as if to the doctor, smiling and saying: "I would like a home birth." Then pause and listen attentively, imagining your doctor's reply. Then repeat your statement. Try this ten times. How did you sound and look? Were you inclined to shout or whisper? Did you cross your arms so that you looked on the defensive? It is not only what you say, but how you say it, that is important. Your tone of voice can convey confidence or invite conflict or bullying. Practise saying, "I've decided that I want a home birth" in as many different ways as possible and settle for the tone and low pitch that makes you sound pleasantly assertive and friendly.

66 None of the local GPs were prepared to take me on, and we were summoned to see the chief obstetrician of the area, who underlined that a home birth was out of the question. We politely said that we should have been grateful for expert assistance at the delivery but, since this was not forthcoming, we preferred to take our chances at home. Several weeks later, out of the blue, a letter arrived informing us that three midwives had been assigned to us.

Once you get approval in principle, most doctors will want to know that you will agree to be transferred to hospital if there are signs that the baby is over-stressed. You can make it clear that you agree to this, provided that everything is explained to you and you don't feel that any decisions are being taken over your head. You may want to say that there are obviously situations in which this would be your choice too, but that you would not want to transfer to hospital just because labour was long drawn-out. Be sure to keep copies of all correspondence concerning your request for a home birth.

For a woman who is disabled, home may be the best place because it is familiar, and she can feel free in a setting that she knows well and which is adapted to her needs. A woman with polyarthritis says, "A lot of disabled women are told, 'You're disabled, so of course you go into hospital.' You don't get any choice at all. But I'm assertive—when you've been in a wheelchair for two years, you know how to get your own way." She was firm that she wanted a home birth and a birthing pool, and found this the ideal solution. "Water encourages you to relax when you're disabled, and you're much freer in water. I just floated, with my boyfriend in the pool supporting me from behind. When we needed the midwives, they were there. When we wanted to be alone, we could be alone." She gave birth to a baby who rotated from the posterior position just before delivery, she had an intact perineum, and her baby was vigorously healthy and alert from the moment of birth.

66 When you have a home birth, you don't have to go to someone else's place. It's your place. That makes all the difference.

Be *assertive*

If your doctor proposes a 'compromise' solution—that you go into hospital for a short time and return home after a few hours, or are booked for a birth room, or suggests that care is modified to meet your special requests about not having drugs, or that electronic fetal monitoring will be used for only 20 minutes or so after you are admitted, and then you will be free to move around—and if you are not happy with that proposed compromise, say so and openly restate what you want.

> You can take time to think about your decision…
> Just say: "I'd like a few days to consider that."

On the other hand you may not want to say 'yes' or 'no' on the spot, and you can take time to think about it, discuss it with your partner, and then write to the doctor if you say, "I'd like a few days to consider that," "We need to talk this through," or "I'll think hard about that and let you know my decision next week." Do not be steamrollered into an agreement that you may regret later.

Having said this, you do not have to put on a perfect performance. You have a right to be emotional, to get angry, to weep, to make mistakes, to be illogical, and even, if that is how it turns out, to be unassertive!

You are entitled to your own ideas about how you would like your birth to be. You are not on trial. You want the best for yourself and your baby. Whatever advice you are given, whatever the strength of other people's feelings, you have the right and responsibility to come to your own informed decision about where you have your baby.

What if my doctor says 'no' to a home birth?

If you come to the decision that you want to give birth at home, this is your right in the UK. The NHS Trust has a legal responsibility to provide appropriate care. If your GP is not happy with your decision, you can change your doctor, or be cared for by a midwife. You also have the right to decline medical intervention of any kind. The introduction of the provisions of the European Convention on Human Rights in 1988[7] makes consent a matter of human rights and in the words of a Professor of Medical Law "respect of bodily integrity and privacy are values that are central to any theory of consent."[8]

Handling stress and keeping a cool head

It is sometimes stated that home birth is safe in the Netherlands because of careful selection. This is true. But it is selection of high risk women for hospital, rather than selection for home birth. In Holland birth is treated as a normal process that can take place at home unless there are special reasons why a woman is advised to go to hospital.

In other countries selection is made for home birth and it is taken for granted that birth takes place in hospital unless a woman shows no deviation from a medically agreed and often rigidly defined idea of 'normal' down to the last detail. Any woman wanting a home birth has to pass a series of examinations to prove herself worthy of it. The testing is itself highly stressful. It may contribute to raised blood pressure and other stress related illnesses, and certainly will increase the woman's anxiety levels. It is very difficult for even the most confident woman to take these examinations in her stride. So it is important to have strong support from someone close (a confiding friend with whom you can share your anxieties), to develop assertiveness skills in dealing with medical encounters and to obtain the knowledge on which you can make informed choices between alternatives from a birth organisation, midwifery and medical journals, books and the Internet. There are more suggestions on the next page.

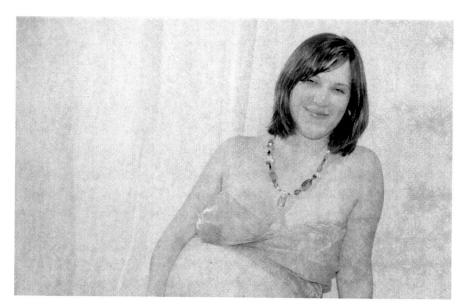

How to handle stress

You will no doubt have your own ways of dealing with stress, but useful approaches include meditation, relaxation, rhythmic, controlled breathing, yoga, energetic physical activity, and creative work. In other words, to reduce your stress levels do anything that helps you feel in control of your life and positive about your pregnancy. Here are a few other suggestions in case you find yourself wondering how to battle through:

♥ Encourage your partner or someone else who is close to you to give you loving support. Tell him or her that you need to have your confidence built up again!

♥ Find a friend in whom you can confide your worries, who is not judgemental.

♥ Use relaxation and massage. You may find aromatherapy oils helpful too.

♥ Meditate and create positive fantasies about your upcoming birth.

♥ Try yoga. You may find a special class for pregnancy in your area.

♥ Do some rhythmic breathing, not as an exercise, but at any time when you are feeling under stress.

♥ Do some physical activity—take a walk, go swimming, do some gardening or go cycling.

♥ Make something. Any kind of creative activity is good. Try making pictures or pots. Or do something which requires creative thinking, such as gardening, baking... Or make some beautiful things for your baby.

♥ Develop some assertiveness skills so as to improve your relationships. Ask your antenatal teacher for guidance and perhaps also request that you do some role-play in class together.

♥ Get some accurate, evidence-based information from well-researched books and research papers. If you have access to the Internet, visit useful sites and get as much information as you can. (See 'Useful contacts' on page 293.)

Get some accurate, evidence-based information from well-researched books and research papers, or from the Internet

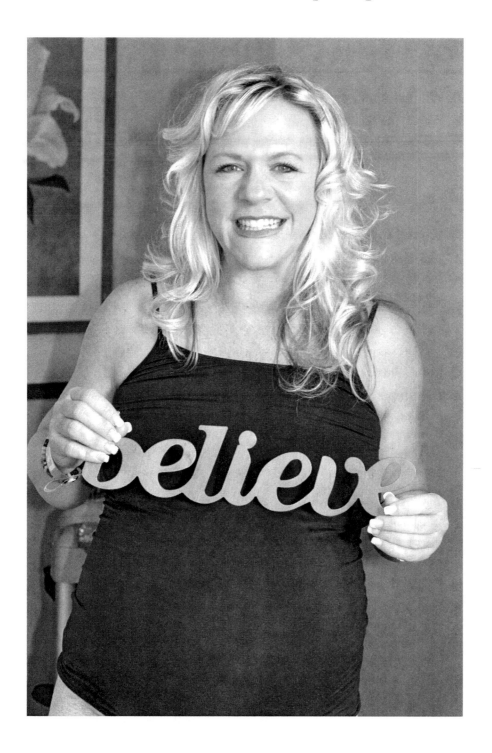

Home birth Q&A:

Q: What should I do to get a home birth?

A. Tell your GP that you want one and contact a home birth support group. The situation varies around the country. (Also see Useful contacts on page 293.)

*Contact a home birth support group.
The situation varies around the country.*

Q: What if my GP discourages me?

A: You have the right to give birth at home. If the GP disapproves he or she should refer you to another GP who supports home births and has midwives attached to the practice.

You have the right to give birth at home

Q: Must I have a hospital doctor at my home birth?

A: A community midwife experienced in home birth is the most appropriate professional caregiver. Consultants and other members of obstetric teams do not attend home births. Most obstetricians have never seen one and only meet women when pregnancy or labour is not straightforward or something has gone wrong and they need hospital treatment.

Q: How do I get antenatal care?

A: Discuss this with your midwife. It is often shared between the GP and the midwife.

Q: How can I arrange a home birth privately?

A: Book an independent midwife. Don't leave it till the last minute. It is best if you get to know each other early so you get continuity of care through pregnancy, labour and after the birth. To find an independent midwife, contact the Independent Midwives Association (see Useful contacts.).

If your GP refuses he or she should refer you to another GP who supports home births and has midwives attached to the practice

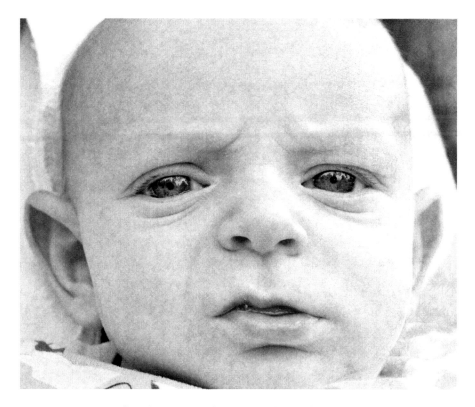

Am I prepared to negotiate the care
I believe is right for me and my baby?

Be strong!

You may find it difficult to arrange the birth you want. Before you start, consider:

- ♥ Can I summon up the stamina, courage and persistence to overcome obstacles that are likely to be put in my way?

- ♥ Where can I obtain the emotional support and practical help from other people that I will need?

- ♥ Am I prepared to be assertive, to state what I want, avoiding both aggression and submission.

- ♥ Am I prepared to negotiate the care I believe is right for me and my baby?

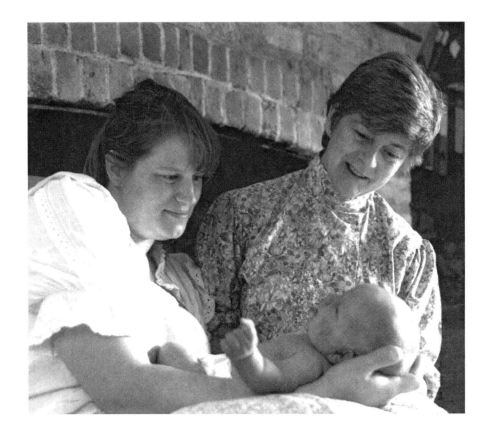

Your midwife

A midwife is quite distinct from a nurse, although midwives have often trained as nurses before training as midwives. In some countries such as the UK, the Netherlands, Denmark and France, there is 'direct entry' for midwives. They do not have to be nurses first, but go straight into midwifery education. In other countries, such as Australia, they must be nurses first. Britain has a mix of nurse-midwives and direct-entry midwives. Direct entry ensures that a midwife's main focus is on birth as a normal life event, rather than a disease and malfunction.

THE ROLE OF MIDWIVES

We are lucky to have midwives in the UK. There is a handful of countries with no organised midwifery system at all: Panama, El Salvador, Venezuela, Colombia, Honduras, the Dominican Republic and Burundi. Alone of all Western industrialised countries, Canada has been without a legal midwifery system of any kind until fairly recently, but now midwifery is recognised and professional training has been developed in Ontario, British Columbia, Alberta and Manitoba.

We are lucky to have midwives in the UK

Midwives are practitioners in their own right and they are the only people whose training is concerned solely with caring for women in childbirth. Consultants (obstetricians) are first and foremost gynaecologists, and their status comes from this rather than from baby-catching. Any doctor is legally allowed to deliver babies, even those with no special training for childbirth. Indeed, in a modern hospital many doctors—even those with obstetric training—have never had a chance to see a birth without intervention of any kind, since even in straightforward labours interventions such as artificial rupture of the membranes, withholding food and fluids from women, and the use of intravenous drips are standard practices. This situation is likely to continue because some doctors see their involvement with childbirth as limited to dealing with abnormalities and complications.

In some countries, such as Britain, midwives have a statutory duty to attend a woman in childbirth when called, wherever the mother is, although they also have to obey instructions from their employers. This puts them in a difficult position. It is a woman's right to give birth where she chooses, and she does not need to book with a doctor for maternity care. Nor does she require a doctor's permission to give birth at home. However, she, or someone else on her behalf, must summon midwife help once labour is underway, or as soon as possible after the birth.

It is a woman's right to give birth where she chooses, and she does not need to book with a doctor for maternity care. Nor does she require a doctor's permission to give birth at home.

Traditional midwifery

Midwives have a long history of persecution going back to the Middle Ages, when many were burned as witches. In North America the midwives who arrived with the waves of migration in the 19th century came to be dismissed as relics of an outmoded lifestyle. There was the feeling that migrants should turn their backs on European traditions in childbirth and favour modern medicine instead. In the UK too, with the advent of the National Health Service after World War II and sudden free access to maternity care in seemingly clean and comfortable hospitals, there was a sudden shift towards hospital care. Therefore, whereas in the early years of the 20th century most women were cared for in their own homes by midwives and family doctors, by the 1940s this had changed to hospital care by doctors, with nurses doing the minor tasks. In remote areas, where few doctors wanted to work, midwifery continued to be practised. The 1970s saw a rebirth of midwifery in the UK and North America, against strong medical opposition.

In some countries and even in some states in the USA, it is against the law for a midwife to attend a birth. To do so is a radical act. (If insurance is required, by law, and insurance is not available, midwifery effectively becomes illegal.) In these cases, there is underground midwifery and midwives constantly risk imprisonment for practising medicine without a licence. If a baby dies, the midwife who was in attendance is tried for manslaughter or even murder. While some states in the USA now register or license midwives, in others the practice of midwifery is still illegal.

Many doctors in North America oppose midwifery because they believe it is dangerous and it threatens their profession and their incomes. They are of the opinion that midwifery offers mothers sub-standard care: "Why settle for a Ford when you can have a Cadillac?" They see themselves as the Cadillacs of birth. It is only in North America, and in hospitals elsewhere based on the American model, that obstetric nurses are used in place of midwives, and that the word 'midwife' suggests outdated care by old grannies.

Actually, some of those granny midwives were very good. There is much that we can learn from the traditional practice of midwifery in rural areas, not only in North America, but anywhere in the world where women healers are part of a long tradition of helping women through the biological transitions of their lives. These caregivers assist not only at each person's coming to birth, but also at the surrendering of life.

A midwife:

---

66 The great advantage of home birth is that the labour is undisturbed. The woman does not have to be moved, and the surroundings are familiar. I don't have all the paperwork that I must do in hospital, and we are all more relaxed.

Midwifery today

The modern, professionally trained midwife is a specialist in childbearing, qualified to take responsibility for women antenatally, through the birth itself, and for four weeks afterwards. She possesses specific skills to support the physiological processes, understands deviations from the norm, and knows when obstetric advice or assistance is required. Unlike a consultant, the main focus of a midwife's interest is the normal, not the pathological, and the whole woman rather than one organ, the uterus. Midwives working outside hospital resort to intervention less readily than hospital midwives because events that would be considered abnormal according to the paradigm of standard hospital labour are considered normal away from the rigid protocols of the hospital.

Hospital midwives have tended to become subordinate members of teams headed by obstetricians, and have been powerless to prevent this. They are used to controlling people waiting in the antenatal clinic, to doing menial jobs such as weighing women and putting a stick in a urine sample to note whether or not it changes colour, to chaperoning doctors when they do a vaginal examination, to preparing equipment for the obstetrician so that he or she can perform an intervention in labour; they are used to cleaning up afterwards, to keeping records, and in some countries where there are too many doctors— such as Italy—to being the doctor's assistant at the birth. Sweden and the Netherlands, both countries with very few baby deaths, are notable exceptions to this trend, and there midwives have retained their professional integrity, with nearly all of the Swedish midwives working in hospitals, but most Dutch midwives doing home births.

In Sweden and the Netherlands midwives have retained their professional integrity—working either at home or in hospitals

A woman has to be very sure a home birth is what she wants

❝ As a midwife I would never persuade a woman to have a home birth. She's got to be very sure that it's what she wants. But I am certain that the majority of complications arise purely because women are in hospital.

A doctor:

❝ I have learnt most about birth from midwives.

Some midwives like being absorbed into hospital systems and do not want more responsibility. Others feel that the freedom to exercise their skills has been eroded. In hospitals women are often seen by junior doctors who are learning about obstetrics. These junior doctors make decisions about care which might be very different from those made by an experienced midwife. Many midwives feel that interventionist procedures are being carried out unnecessarily by some of the senior doctors and obstetricians.

So midwives are in a difficult position. Some opt for security in a hospital system and do not step out of line. Others fight that system from the inside. Still others decide to serve women outside hospital and attend home births and work in birth centres although, to do this, they may have to become independent, private midwives. (In most countries this means working separately from the standard health service.) In the Netherlands independent midwifery is the norm and midwives are on a professional par with general practitioners. About 70% of them work outside hospitals and 16% in hospitals. (The rest are in clinics, midwifery schools, doing research, and so on.) In Italy, by contrast, the vast majority work in hospitals and only a handful are independent. For most Italian women, except those in cities such as Florence, Rome, Genoa, and Turin, who are seeking home birth in increasing numbers, it is a sign of poverty to go to a midwife.[1] You can find out about independent midwives from the organisations listed in 'Useful contacts' on page 293.

In the Netherlands independent midwifery is the norm

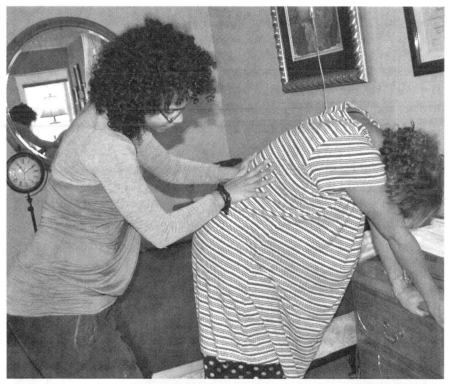

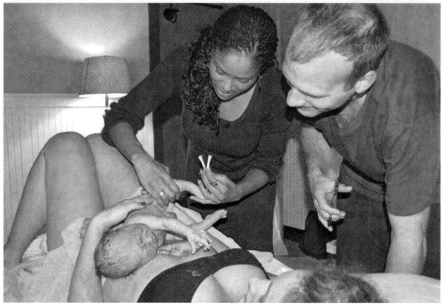

THE MIDWIFE AND HOME BIRTH

For a midwife who has worked only in hospitals, it can be threatening to take on a home birth. The worst mistake she can make is to try to 'move hospital to the home' and attempt to practise exactly as she would in hospital. She needs to think through how she is going to support the woman so that there is the greatest chance of labour progressing naturally at its own pace and in its own way.

66 All midwives are based at our hospital... When I started labour, my husband had to go and fetch the midwives from the hospital (I suppose they were without cars). On his arrival the Night Sister greeted him with "Couldn't you persuade her to come in? It would be much safer."

66 It was good to be at home but, if there can be such a thing, it was a hospitalised home confinement. They turned our bedroom into a hospital. Everything was timed, recorded, methodical, sterile.

A midwife's responsibilities

Anxiety is contaminating. Anyone who is apprehensive around a woman in labour communicates his or her own fear, and can have a negative effect on the labour. It is the responsibility of the midwife to face up to and explore her fears well in advance of attending a home birth and to share them with colleagues who have experience of working outside hospital, so that she does not bring infectious anxiety with her to a birth. It helps if she has already attended births outside hospital as an assistant to an experienced midwife.

When a midwife attends in quiet confidence, she is able to tolerate inaction and can watch and wait on this child's coming to life, sharing with the mother her own strength and inner joy.

When a midwife attends in quiet confidence, she is able to tolerate inaction and can watch and wait on the child's coming

Who makes a good midwife?

♥ A good midwife blends with the surroundings, merging with the pattern of that woman's life. She does not take charge or take over. She does not "manage" labour. Her task is more difficult than this. It demands great strength of personality. She observes minutely and with sensitive awareness everything that is happening in the labour and is aware of what is happening in the mind of the woman she is attending.

> A good midwife blends with the surroundings,
> merging with the pattern of that woman's life

♥ A baby may weigh three kilos or five kilos and still be of normal birth weight. In the same way a labour can be completely normal and yet be far from average. Dilation may be slow or very rapid. The woman may have an overwhelming desire to push or almost none at all. Expulsion may take 10 minutes or four hours. There may be lulls and rest phases. Each labour has its rhythm, its own cadences, which make it different from all others.

♥ A good midwife understands when she should stand back and let things unfold and she knows when she needs to intervene. And interventions are rare. Far more often she gives quiet, tender support to the woman in her care, simply allowing the energy of birth to sweep through the mother's body, and helping her to find strength within herself. When you see a river in full flood, you know that you cannot fight its power. But you can use it so that its flow sweeps you onwards.

♥ A woman should be able to expect open and honest communication with the midwife. Instead of "reassurance" there is frank explanation, exploring of options, a genuine sharing between the two women, which goes far beyond the trite phrases that are sometimes trotted out in an attempt to keep a patient docile and placid.

♥ When a woman and her midwife relate to each other with mutual respect, warmth and openness, it is as if they are on a journey together in which exciting discoveries are made. Their understanding deepens and they are both enriched by the birth experience.

♥ A good midwife loves women. She does not dominate, direct, or even instruct. The word 'midwife' is Anglo-Saxon for 'with woman'. The midwife is side by side and with the woman. Except on the rare occasions when she needs to take decisive action to avert danger, she follows rather than leads. Ina May Gaskin, spiritual midwife at The Farm, the alternative-style community in Tennessee, says, "Pregnant and birthing mothers are elemental forces, in the same way that gravity, thunderstorms, earthquakes, and hurricanes are elemental forces. In order to understand the laws of their energy flow, you have to love and respect them for their magnificence, at the same time that you study them with the accuracy of a true scientist."[2]

♥ A good midwife does not criticise or judge the woman in her care, and even though a woman may be submissive and seek approval, she helps her stand on her own feet and to find the locus of control inside herself.

A good midwife does not criticise or judge the woman in her care

♥ When women give birth in hospital, they often apologise to their midwives. Professor Mavis Kirkham wrote of a hospital research project: "Most of the women I observed in labour apologised. Many apologised frequently if they felt they were not behaving well or were 'being a nuisance', or 'causing trouble' by making requests, or simply receiving routine care from busy staff. The commonest words I heard women say immediately after delivery were "I'm sorry..."[3] When women placate authority in this way, their deference is implicit acknowledgement of an institutional power structure in which they are at the lowest level. They are, in effect, intruders on the professional territory of the hospital. If midwives accept these apologies, they, too, acknowledge and submit to this power structure.

♥ A good midwife is not only someone who delivers a baby. She is midwife to a woman's transformation to motherhood and a man's transformation to fatherhood. She is midwife to all the dreams and hopes surrounding the coming to being of that child, and to the process of maturing and growth that is involved for both parents.

A midwife facilitates a woman's transformation to motherhood

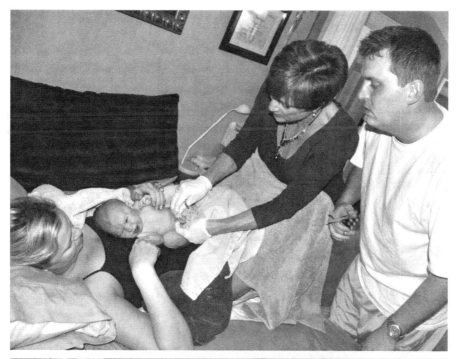

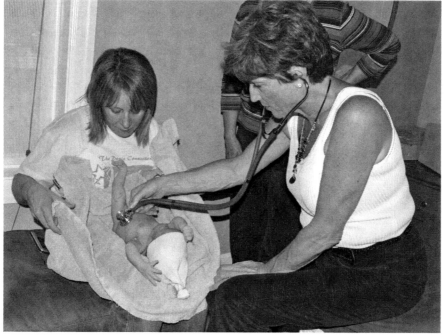

Meeting your midwife

Even though midwifery is the foundation of care in childbirth throughout Europe, and the whole system would collapse if midwives walked out, most countries no longer provide any continuity of care. Different groups of midwives work in the antenatal clinic, the labour and delivery rooms, and on the postpartum ward. At a time in their lives when women are at their most vulnerable, they meet total strangers. In Britain attempts are being made—through the creation of midwife teams who get to know the mothers in their care during pregnancy—to deal with this problem of anonymity, which is frustrating and often confusing for midwives, as well as mothers. But only in Denmark and the Netherlands is it the norm to have continuity of care from your own midwife. In southern Europe doctors have totally taken over antenatal care, and even in countries where midwife care at birth is the normal system, a woman who is having her baby in hospital may never meet the midwives assigned to her until she is admitted in labour. Having your baby outside hospital may be your only opportunity to get to know your midwife.

Questions to ask

At your first meetings with your midwife, or with the small group of midwives who are attending you, there will be many questions to ask. If you are choosing an independent midwife, you will need to put these questions before you can come to a firm arrangement with each other. Either way, you won't want to fire questions at her, but you can incorporate many of these into your discussion with her. Here are some of the questions that you may like to bear in mind:

♥ How long have you been a midwife?

♥ Why did you become a midwife?

♥ What was your training?

♥ How many mothers have you attended and, of these, how many were home births or not in a large hospital?

♥ Do you work with other midwives?

♥ What happens if two women you have booked are in labour at the same time?

♥ Will I be able to meet your colleagues?

♥ What is your back-up system? Do you work with any doctors?

♥ What equipment do you carry with you? Do you carry any drugs for pain relief and to stimulate the uterus?

♥ What resuscitation equipment do you carry for the baby?

♥ What antenatal care do you provide? Are there any home visits?

♥ Do you offer childbirth classes or pregnancy discussion groups? If not, which classes do you recommend?

♥ What postnatal care do you provide?

♥ What do you do if a woman has a very long labour?

♥ What is the plan of action if transfer to hospital should be necessary?

♥ Under what conditions do you transfer and what are your transfer rates?

♥ [If she works in a birth centre, midwifery-led unit or GP unit] Are there any standard procedures that must be followed regarding admission and when I am in labour, such as compulsory fetal monitoring, birth positions, etc?

♥ What are your views on routine episiotomy? What is your episiotomy rate?

♥ How often do your mothers have an intact perineum?

♥ What happens if my perineum requires suturing? Will you do this yourself or call a doctor?

♥ When are your holidays? If you plan to go on holiday towards the end of my pregnancy or within three weeks after I am due, and I go into labour, who should I call?

66 She was wonderful... She visited me at home in the early stages of my pregnancy, and chatted as a friend would over a cup of coffee... As my pregnancy progressed, she called at the house once a week for her own personal check-up. She made friends with my 3-year-old, letting her feel my tummy and listen to the baby's heartbeat.

Points to consider

You may want to discuss the following issues with your midwife:

- ♥ nutrition in pregnancy

- ♥ who you would like with you at the birth

- ♥ fetal monitoring

- ♥ moving around during labour

- ♥ positions for birth

- ♥ using a birth pool

- ♥ exactly what help she gives a mother to avoid the need for episiotomy

- ♥ her basic beliefs about birth and breastfeeding

- ♥ what exactly you are hoping for with this birth

If you are booking an independent midwife, you will also want to ask her fee, when it should be paid, and what is included.

After you have met, one of the most important questions of all for *you* to answer is whether you like her as a person and feel relaxed and confident with her. Can you be completely open about how you feel and what you want? Talk with other women for whom she has cared to find out about their experience with her. You can learn a great deal from them.

> After you have met your midwife, one of the most important questions is whether you like her as a person and feel relaxed

Any woman who chooses to become a midwife cares deeply for other women and loves babies. Yet midwives working in hospitals have often learnt to guard their feelings and have been forced to hold back from giving themselves completely. They have been warned not to 'become emotionally involved with the patient'. When a midwife works in a different environment, outside the rigid hospital system, she is free to be herself and to have a close, caring relationship with a woman whom she comes to know, not as a patient, but as a sister.

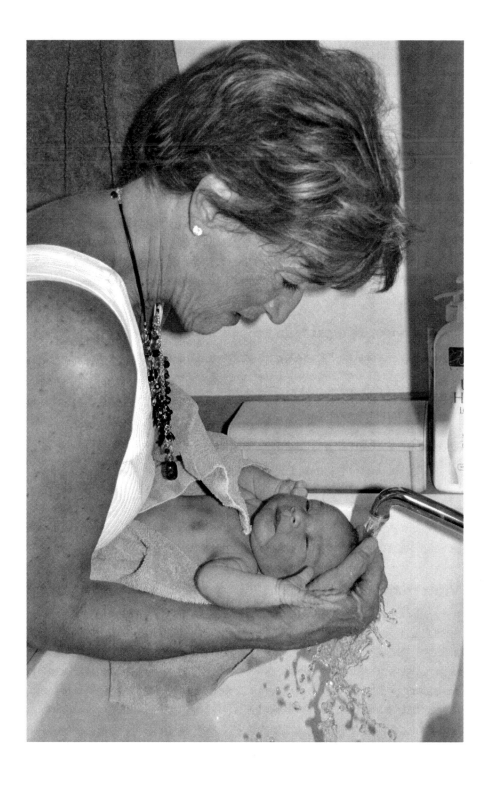

The role of the midwife Q&A:

Q: How are midwives different from consultants?

A: Unlike consultants, the main focus of the care midwives offer is the normal, not the pathological, and the whole woman rather than one organ, the uterus. A good midwife knows how to keep birth normal.

Q: What does a midwife do?

A: A midwife is a specialist in childbearing, qualified to take responsibility for women antenatally, through the birth itself, and for four weeks afterwards. She has specific skills to support the physiological process, understands deviations from the norm, and knows when obstetric advice or assistance is required.

Q: How is this different from hospital?

A: Hospital midwives often become subordinate members of teams headed by obstetricians, and they have been powerless to prevent this. Some opt for the security in a hospital system and do not step out of line. Others fight the system from the inside.

Q: Is it important that I like my midwife?

A: One of the most important questions of all for you to answer is whether you like your midwife as a person and feel relaxed and confident with her. Can you be completely open about how you feel and what you want? Talk with other women for whom she has cared to find out about their experience with her. You can learn a great deal from them.

Visits from your midwife

For any woman who only meets her midwife when she is admitted to hospital in labour and who then may find that this person disappears with the next shift change, the experience of bearing a child is bound to be fragmented and depersonalised. However, when a woman gets to know her midwife during pregnancy and the two become friends, a bond of understanding develops and the emotional support the midwife gives can help the mother feel confident and strong.

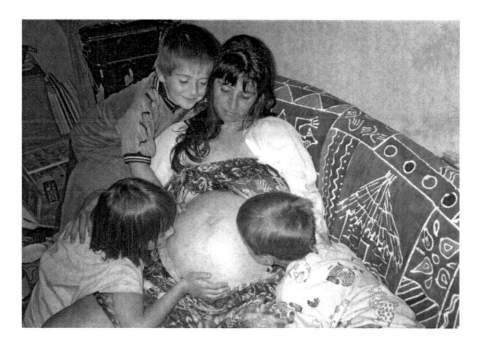

A visit from your midwife is fun for the older child too. He or she will learn about how babies are born in the most natural way possible and will be shown how to feel the firm curve of the baby's bottom. Your older child will probably be delighted when a little foot kicks against his or her hand. The new baby will not come as a surprise or as an alien invader, but as someone who he or she has already learnt about and even touched. Even when your midwife is fixing on a blood pressure cuff and blowing it up, your child will probably feel intrigued. It's likely your midwife will explain what she's doing and she may even let your older child have a go! This kind of relationship with a child is much easier when antenatal care takes place at home. This is because your child will be in a familiar place and on his or her own territory and the midwife will be coming in as a family friend, not as a stranger.

Needless to say, your own experience of midwifery care will also benefit in similar ways because you will be meeting her in your own home, or in a familiar birth centre. Your relationship—which will have developed during your pregnancy—should help you relax during your labour and birth and really trust your midwife and the support she gives you.

Your relationship with your midwife should help you relax during your labour and birth and really trust your midwife

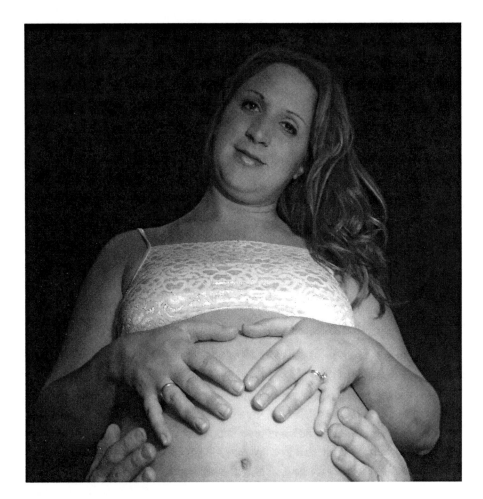

Getting ready

Now that you have made the decision to give birth out of hospital, you can prepare to make it the best experience possible. The chances of a safe, happy birth are enormously increased if you approach labour healthy, energetic, well-nourished, and self-confident, if you learn movements that allow your body to open up, and if you know how to relax and breathe rhythmically.

YOUR ANTENATAL CARE

❝ I have to go on the bus to get to the clinic, as I haven't a car. The journey takes 45 minutes each way, and I usually have to wait at least half an hour. I have two—perhaps three—minutes with the doctor. The only reason I go is because I'd worry that something was going wrong if I didn't.

❝ The midwife came to see me at home and spent a lot of time talking about what I wanted. She became a friend and we all look forward to her visits.

The fragmentation of care that often occurs in hospital clinics results from different staff members performing different tests as women are shuffled from one line of chairs to another, from room to room, from cubicle to cubicle, from person to person.

Yet, even if you escape being screened by a variety of anonymous doctors, nurses, midwives and radiographers, you are still not receiving good antenatal care if you have tests that detract from, or take the place of your caregivers' relationship with you as a unique human being. Antenatal care should be far more than screening for abnormalities. You need holistic care, to be cared for as a whole person, rather than merely tested for potential problems.

Even if a woman has only one caregiver, or a small group of caregivers, the medical model rather than the holistic model of care is often adopted. It entails turning her into a patient and dividing up information about her body so that it can be laid out on a record card: blood pressure, weight, urine, haemoglobin, and height of fundus. Her hopes and fears, the stresses of her daily life, financial worries, conflicts in the family, problems at work—these social and emotional aspects of pregnancy are seen as irrelevant compared with physical symptoms that can be checked, enumerated and recorded.

The fragmentation of care that often occurs in hospital clinics results from different staff members performing different tests

Many unnecessary investigations take place in antenatal clinics today. Some are potentially harmful. Since the early years of the last century, when obstetric-style antenatal care was first introduced, tests have proliferated. Doctors seem to be under the impression that any item of information might come in useful sometime, somehow. But information is useless unless it affects the kind of care that is provided.

Midwives in many traditional cultures were giving antenatal care long before the 20th century, visiting the pregnant woman's home to teach her about pregnancy, to discuss diet, work and exercise, to massage her with oil and palpate her uterus, to talk with her about her husband and family, to ward off danger with shared religious rites and prayers, and to make plans for the birth. Traditional midwives have usually been far more than birth attendants.

66 He said, "The baby's very small, you know. Try and eat more." Next time I saw another doctor, who told me, "You've got a good-sized baby there. It's going to be a whopper!" I don't know what to believe. Should I be stuffing myself to try and make the baby bigger or will it be so huge that it can't get out?

66 It was a shambles really. The doctor gave me the wrong card. It was a different blood group, and it said 'Rhesus negative' but I am Rhesus positive. I didn't realise till much later, but I could have had a whole lot of treatment I didn't need, and the other woman, who had my card, wouldn't have had treatment that she needed. At least they let us keep our own records. If the clinic had kept them, it might never have been found out.

Today obstetricians construct the agenda for antenatal care. As we have seen already, there is strong evidence that other influences on pregnant women—socio-economic conditions that result in inequalities in health—usually have more effect on the outcome of pregnancy than anything that the most dedicated of obstetricians can do in an antenatal clinic. Socially deprived women, who are most in need of care, are most likely to delay seeking it.

A woman with a 10-month-old baby and a two-and-a-half-year-old child, no help at home, nobody else to care for the children, and no private transport, may find it difficult to attend an antenatal clinic even though it is only two or three miles away. A teenager who is hoping against hope that she is not pregnant, trying to hide it from her family, and with no idea of how to get help, is unlikely to find her way to the antenatal clinic until pregnancy is well-advanced.

It is much safer to have a baby if you are educated and well-off than if you are uneducated and poor. In England and Wales perinatal mortality rates are worked out on the basis of the husband's occupation. Twice as many babies die in Social Class 5, at the bottom of the scale, as in Social Class 1, at the top.[1]

Standard antenatal care entails up to 15 visits to a clinic or hospital, or a mixture of both, and a woman may encounter 50 or more different professionals, many of whom make conflicting comments and give contradictory advice. Far from providing reassurance, these encounters increase anxiety.

Routine antenatal tests

There is no point in having tests unless their results are going to affect care. Useless information provided by routine tests is often employed as a charm against a perilous passage, in the same way that talismans have been used traditionally by pregnant women to guard against evil. With modern antenatal care this information is often not even conveyed to the mother, but is retained by the doctor and recorded, as part of a series of illegible hieroglyphs resembling mystic runes, in case notes that are sometimes not even passed on to other caregivers.

The results of most tests have a margin of error that's often wide

The results of most tests have a margin of error that is often wide and can lead to false negative and false positive diagnoses. False negative diagnosis suggests that there is no problem when in fact there is one. False positive diagnosis appears to reveal a problem when there is none. Both are dangerous. The first gives rise to complacency in the face of special risk. The second causes needless anxiety, and may lead to unnecessary interventions, such as induction of labour or caesarean section.

How antenatal tests may lead to a chain of interventions:

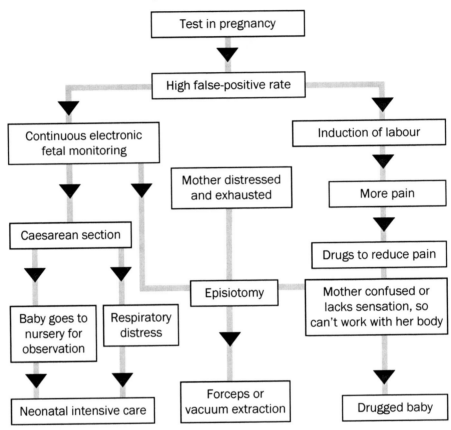

Here are some tests which you can safely avoid:

- There is nothing gained from regularly testing urine for sugar in pregnancy unless you are diabetic. A trace of sugar in urine is very common. It may simply mean that you have recently eaten something especially sweet. Bananas sometimes have this effect.

- Routine weighing is a waste of time too. Weight checks give useful information only if you started pregnancy very underweight or very overweight. The baby's growth is better assessed by having one or two caregivers regularly palpate your uterus so that they are in touch, literally, with the baby's development.

- Vaginal examinations in pregnancy are usually unnecessary. In some countries, including the USA, they are performed weekly starting at 37 weeks. In Britain one vaginal examination is often done routinely some time between 33 and 37 weeks. However, vaginal examinations increase the risk of infection and premature rupture of the membranes and, because of this, caesarean section.[2]

Vaginal examinations in pregnancy are usually unnecessary

- Ultrasound enables obstetricians to visualise the baby in the uterus and learn much more about fetal development, and it reveals certain abnormalities. If you have a scan at around 16 weeks, both the date of conception and the expected date of delivery can be estimated fairly accurately, but only within two weeks. If you are unsure about the date you conceived, you might decide that this is a good reason for choosing to have a scan. If you have already had a low birth weight baby, you may also want to monitor fetal growth with several ultrasound scans. However, diagnosis of the baby's weight based on fundal height is almost as accurate as that from ultrasound, so whether or not you have a series of scans is up to you.[3]

- Biochemical tests of fetal wellbeing proliferated in the 70s and 80s. They included alpha-fetaprotein testing, measurement of hCG (human chorionic gonadotrophin), placental proteins, hPL (human placental lactogen) and oestrogen levels with 24-hour urine specimens, blood tests, or, occasionally, measurement of levels in the saliva. A small proportion of the biochemical tests available can be useful in early pregnancy to screen for abnormalities. But tests later in pregnancy to try to predict low birth weight, premature birth or stillbirth are a waste of time.[4]

- Cardiotocography—fetal heart rate monitoring in pregnancy—has added to obstetricians' knowledge about life inside the uterus. However, four randomised controlled trials have not demonstrated any direct benefit for mothers and babies. So you may decide that it is not worth having this.[5]

Research has not shown any direct benefit for mothers or babies in carrying out fetal heart rate monitoring in pregnancy

Holistic antenatal care

If you are having holistic antenatal care, you will be offered only those screening procedures that are likely to give useful information and make a difference in the care that is given during pregnancy or at the birth. While being alert to the possibility of pathology, its main focus is woman-centred. It enables you to care for yourself, instead of just being at the receiving end of care. It is concerned with feelings and relationships that are important to you rather than merely with physiology. And it helps you grow in self-awareness, self-confidence and strength. Holistic antenatal care is empowering.

For care to be holistic, it is essential to have a continuing relationship with a few caregivers only, who get to know you well and who make time at each visit to obtain full and accurate information. You talk freely, in a totally accepting atmosphere. There is genuine sharing.

THE BEST POSSIBLE DIET

When you conceive and in the first eight weeks of pregnancy, it is important to have a diet rich in folic acid. This is present in dark green leafy vegetables, whole grains, yeast and nuts. It is in liver, too, but it is easy to get too much Vitamin A from liver and that is toxic. It is a good idea to take supplementary folic acid if you are likely to get pregnant and in early pregnancy when rapid cell division is taking place and the baby's spinal cord and brain is forming.

Everything you eat during pregnancy should enhance your feeling of wellbeing and be good for you and the baby. Choose wholegrain bread and cereals, fruit and vegetables—freshly picked whenever you can get them. To ensure a good supply of Vitamin C have one raw fruit or vegetable meal every day. Eat some protein at each meal, either in the form of meat, fish, dairy products (such as cheese, milk, eggs—thoroughly cooked—and yoghurt), a soya bean product such as tofu, or a mix of pulses (peas, beans or lentils) and grains (bread, rice or pasta). Eat iron-rich foods; leafy green vegetables and egg yolks are good sources. Use olive oil, sunflower oil and other polyunsaturated oils as a large proportion of your fats, and enjoy the sugar in fresh and dried fruit, rather than adding sugar to desserts.

An excess of any one type of food is bad. It is possible, for example, to have carrot poisoning, and even to die of it. People have had coronaries associated with eating, among other things, excessive quantities of meat and dairy foods.

When considering your diet in pregnancy, think about the foods you enjoy most. It may be a good idea to write them down. Then look at what you have written to see if any of them do not measure up to your standards of nutrition. Are there any junk foods? Do they contain artificial colourings or are they full of preservatives? Do any provide empty calories? Are there too many fatty foods? If you are particularly fond of food which you know is not good for you, you might then list what you especially like about it: salty, crunchy, crisp, sweet, smooth, filling, quick to make, cheap, reminds me of home (or Rome, or Vienna, or somewhere else). Invariably, there are alternatives that bring a similar sense of wellbeing.

When you look at what you enjoy about the foods that are not so good for you, think how you can find the same qualities in more nutritious foods. If you want an instant food, choose a bowl of nuts and raisins, bite into a banana or apple, or bake a potato in the microwave. If you long for something hot and satisfying, a pan of homemade soup heated up on the stove is more nutritious and probably tastier and more satisfying than a mug of hot chocolate—although you need not rule out the hot chocolate entirely.

At the end of pregnancy many women become constipated and this can be treated by eating more wholegrain bread and muesli. But this is effective only if you also cut your fat intake to the minimum.

In an overview of all the studies of nutrition in pregnancy, the head of the epidemiology programme at the Human Nutrition Research Center on Ageing at Tuft's University in Massachusetts concludes: "There can be no rational justification for allowing pregnant women to go hungry or for imposing either dietary restrictions or marked manipulation of the dietary constituents upon them."[7] So relax and enjoy your food!

Salt in pregnancy

Despite the advice often given to omit salt in order to prevent pre-eclampsia, there is no convincing evidence that salt restriction is effective in achieving this. A study of 2,000 pregnant women, half of whom were recommended to increase salt, and the other half to avoid it, revealed that there were significantly fewer women with pre-eclampsia in the high-salt group. Nor do you need to force yourself to eat large quantities of high-protein foods, since an excessive amount of protein can reduce a baby's birth weight.[6]

MEDICATION & SUPPLEMENTS

You will know already that it is wise to avoid drugs in pregnancy unless you really need them. But there can be few hard and fast rules, and it is usually a question of weighing up the risks and benefits of the drug against the risks and benefits of not treating a disease. Sometimes a pregnant woman has an illness that holds possible dangers for the baby. Then, treating the illness is a sensible choice, even though it entails taking a drug. A high fever, for example, can cause miscarriage and, if the fever can't be brought down in any other way, it is probably better to take paracetamol.

With drugs you usually need to weigh up risks and benefits

All dietary supplements, including vitamins and minerals, are drugs and the system may become overloaded with one mineral or vitamin, which results in nutritional deficiency. Some supplements—such as Vitamins A and D—are toxic in high doses. So avoid mega-vitamins and, unless you know that you suffer from nutritional deficiencies that cannot be rectified by a change of diet, do not take supplementary vitamins and minerals, other than folic acid and other B vitamins.

Herbs, etc

A drug is not necessarily safe for pregnancy because it occurs naturally in the wild. Herbs are powerful and they can be poisonous. Most herbs prescribed by reputable herbalists—select one who is a member of an association of registered practitioners of alternative or complementary medicine—are safe. But others may be teratogenic (cause congenital malformation), or lead to miscarriage. The following herbs are potentially dangerous for anyone, whether pregnant or not: comfrey, berberis, ragwort and prickly ash. Excessive intake of ginseng, feverfew and the kernels of apricots, plums and peaches can also be harmful.

Some herbs increase uterine muscle tone, so can be helpful in producing effective contractions in labour. But the same herbs used in pregnancy, in high doses and by women who are particularly vulnerable, may be associated with miscarriage. So it is wise to avoid herbs such as feverfew and pennyroyal.[8]

Supplements

If you are healthy, you are unlikely to need iron supplements. An increased blood supply in pregnancy results in dilution of haemoglobin and this often causes a normal drop in haemoglobin levels. This is a natural process that helps the flow of blood across the placenta to the baby. In fact it is a sign of fetal wellbeing. If your haemoglobin level does not fall beneath 9.5 grams per decilitre, there is no need for iron supplements).[9] Unnecessary iron supplementation can cause constipation that results in piles, and may result in macrocytosis, where red blood cells enlarge and become sticky so that they cannot flow through fine capillaries, impairing circulation. Also, very high haemoglobin levels in pregnancy are associated with low birth weight. So there is a disadvantage in artificially boosting your haemoglobin level unless you are anaemic.[10]

> It is in the interest of pharmaceutical companies
> to sell their supplements as widely as possible

It is in the interest of pharmaceutical companies who manufacture vitamin and mineral supplements to sell them as widely as possible and to persuade doctors that their patients need them. There is no reason why any pregnant woman should be dosed with these as a matter of routine, and vitamins and minerals are best obtained from a well-balanced diet with plenty of fresh fruit and vegetables, wholegrain cereals, and protein in the form of milk and milk products, pulses, and—for non-vegetarians—meat and fish.

When a woman's haemoglobin is low, caregivers are concerned that if she loses a lot of blood during or after the birth she will be very weak and ill, and need a blood transfusion. This is one reason why, when haemoglobin levels are low at the end of pregnancy, they may be reluctant to support a woman's wish to have a home birth. It seems sensible to have a blood test at, say, 36 weeks to check the haemoglobin level, so that there is time for any supplementation to take effect, if it is needed. If a woman is still anaemic when labour starts, the third stage of labour can be actively managed with an injection of syntometrine. This reduces blood loss and makes haemorrhage less likely. A midwife at a home birth will feel far more confident if she knows that you are willing to accept this if she considers it necessary.

EXERCISE

Regular exercise that you really enjoy helps you feel positive about your pregnant body, tones your muscles and whips up the circulation. Here are a few notes on specific forms of exercise:

♥ Swimming is excellent, because it is so easy to move when floating in water that takes your weight.

♥ Brisk walking in the countryside or a park is good too.

♥ Many women go to aerobic classes which are specially adapted to pregnancy.

♥ One form of dancing is especially suitable: belly dancing—the slow, sinuous kind, rather than rapid gyrations with a diamond in your navel! Belly dancing was traditionally taught in North Africa as part of fertility rituals to mark a girl's passage to womanhood. Women attending a birth danced while the mother rolled her pelvis in a similar way during contractions. Any movement like this that frees the pelvis can help the baby's head to rotate and descend deep into the pelvis.

♥ Special yoga classes for pregnancy are helpful, since they include opening movements for the pelvis and, at the same time, help you find a focus of concentration inside yourself in a very satisfying way. The result is confidence and inner poise.

♥ Many active birth classes are based on yoga. In these you learn movements to enable muscles to 'give' and help your pelvis widen to let the baby through. You practise a range of upright positions and movements and discover how your partner can support you in different positions during labour. Like yoga, these exercises also lead to improved physical coordination, increased self-confidence and a sense of inner balance.

One of the best things about exercise is the healthy glow and sense of luxurious relaxation that comes afterwards. Give yourself time to enjoy that.

Regular exercise that you really enjoy helps you feel positive about your pregnant body, tones your muscles, and whips up the circulation

Swimming is excellent because it is so easy to move
when floating in water that takes your weight

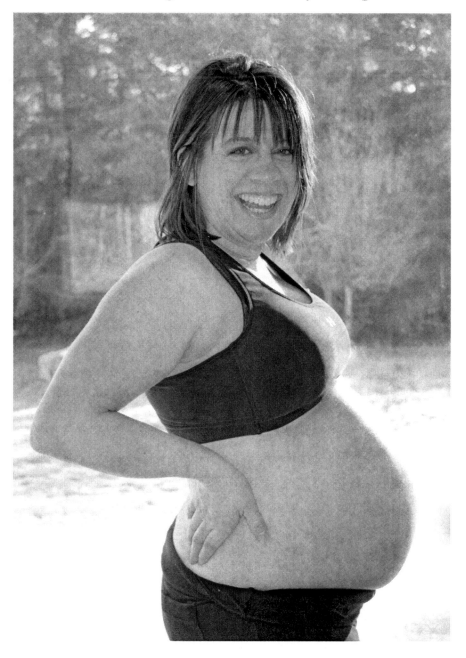

Exercise to avoid

Avoid competitive games, in which you are inclined to ignore the messages of tiredness and pain coming from your body because you are out to beat the other person. It is not a good idea to ignore messages from your body during pregnancy, so these games should be avoided.

If your pelvic ligaments stretch too much in late pregnancy, so that you feel like a disjointed doll, have backache and stumble often, pronounced pelvic movements that entail hollowing your lower back may make things worse. Select only those movements that involve tightening your buttocks and abdominal muscles, gently releasing and then tightening them again.

Yoga Q&A:

Q: How can yoga help in pregnancy?

A: Special yoga classes for pregnancy are useful, since they include opening movements for the pelvis and, at the same time, help you find a focus of concentration inside yourself in a very satisfying way. Yoga also teaches you to breathe rhythmically and fully.

Q: Can yoga actually help me in labour?

A: Yes. Many active birth classes are based on yoga. In these you learn movements to enable muscles to 'give' and help your pelvis widen to let the baby through. You practise a range of upright positions and movements and discover how your partner can support you in different positions during labour.

Q: Does yoga have any other effects?

A: Yoga and active birth classes also lead to improved physical coordination, increased self-confidence and a sense of inner balance.

Q: Is yoga safe for pregnant women?

A: Special yoga classes for pregnancy should be safe, but if any movement proves a strain or causes pain, drop it from the routine and concentrate on easy, flowing, rhythmic movements instead.

Q: Must I have done yoga before?

A: Many classes designed for pregnant women are suitable for complete beginners. Always check this when you book the class.

Q: When can I start yoga classes?

A: You can attend classes from when you are three months pregnant, but again, check this with your yoga teacher.

REST & RELAXATION

You will get the most out of your pregnancy if you can take time to rest and nurture yourself. That means making a space in your life to do anything you like—listen to music, read, dream, or do nothing at all. Find a space where you don't feel under stress to strive to reach a goal, to live up to a standard, or to please someone else.

It is very difficult to do this when you have other children and little or no help with them. It's difficult to do if your partner dismisses domestic work as trivial and something he was never much good at anyway. It's also difficult to do if your job is the kind which consumes all your energy. Your own feelings of responsibility and the guilt you feel when you are not meeting other people's expectations of you may hold you back from creating this small, private citadel of time and space that is yours alone. But if you can do it, you will feel more 'centred' and better able to relax and enjoy being pregnant.

I remember reading a short story in which the heroine was in labour: "I must, I MUST relax!" she muttered fiercely. The feeling that relaxation is compulsory, that if you don't manage to relax, something awful will happen, and that you have to fight to achieve it makes you more tense. Relaxation is a luxury.

If you are having your baby at home or in another out-of-hospital setting, relaxation is the basis of your preparation for birth. It is also a major protection against stress in pregnancy and it is invaluable after the baby comes, when you need to relax in order to breastfeed, as well as to make all the adjustments— the amazing leap across the great divide—entailed in becoming a parent.

Creating a relaxing environment

It helps to have a quiet, peaceful place where you are least likely to be interrupted and where, like an animal in her lair, you can go to ground. It might be your bed, the bath, a garden, a couch in front of an open fire, at the seashore or in a meadow. Any comfortable space where, if only for 10 minutes, you will not be disturbed by the phone ringing or people demanding your attention, will do fine.

First make a nest for yourself with cushions, perhaps a duvet, a beanbag, or some rolled-up towels or rugs. If you are in the bath, slip a small rolled towel behind your neck or use a neck cushion. If you are in a chair, on the ground, or in bed, either recline, well-supported with cushions, or lie down on your side.

In late pregnancy avoid lying flat on your back. In this position your heavy uterus tends to press on the vena cava, the large vein in the lower part of your body. This slows down the blood flow back to your heart and may make you feel sick and giddy, as well as restricting blood flow to the placenta, and oxygen to the baby. So, either sitting well propped-up or lying on your side, support your head and neck with cushions and get comfortable. If you are on your side, a cushion under your upper knee often helps. If you are sitting up, you will need one in the small of your back. The first few times you do this, it is useful to have someone read the following passage for you, slowly, in a low-pitched voice.

♥ Bend your arms and knees and let your body spread, taking as much space as possible. Release tension on a long breath out. Then let the breath flow in when you are ready for it. Don't suck air in. Just allow your lungs to fill. There is a slight pause, as when the crest of a wave is reached, after which you give another breath out, relaxing all down your back and right down to your toes as you do so.

♥ As you listen to the sound of your breathing, be aware of your whole body: your skin where it touches the air and the fabric of your clothing, the strong muscles underneath, your swelling uterus with the baby moving inside it, and the blood pulsing through your body.

♥ Are there any parts of your body that are holding on to tension? You may want to find a more comfortable position. Roll your head slightly forwards and round your shoulders. If you are not completely comfortable, have a stretch and resettle. Or roll into a ball like a hedgehog and then slowly uncurl until you feel at ease.

♥ As you continue to nest, listen to your slow breathing and relax a little more with each breath out. Enjoy your breathing as if you were listening to waves on the seashore. Focus on the breath out and you will find that the breath in looks after itself.

To derive most advantage from relaxation, you need to practise it daily, setting aside a regular time for this self-nurturing. If you have the opportunity, take a rest after lunch or perhaps in the evening when you return from work. But, even if you can do it only when you wake up in the morning or go to bed at night, or if you wake up to empty your bladder and find it difficult to get back to sleep, 10 minutes' relaxation will help you.

BREATHING EXERCISES, OR NOT...

Should you do breathing exercises? You will know how to breathe when you are in labour, just as you know how to breathe now.

Breathing responds instantly to emotions. When we are apprehensive, we breathe jerkily. We hold our breath if we are very afraid, and pain can make us gasp. Under stress some people breathe heavily and quickly, and they hyperventilate. The sensations of hyperventilation are pins and needles in the fingers, numbness around the mouth, and a feeling of dizziness and sickness. Giving birth, even the most beautiful and satisfying birth, is a highly stressful activity so it is understandable that many women overbreathe and hyper-ventilate when contractions are coming thick and fast.

Getting prepared

During your pregnancy get to know your own breathing habits, noticing how your breathing changes with your emotions. If it is difficult to observe this, ask your partner to help. Are there any times when you tend to breathe arhythmically (*not* rhythmically), or are there any times when you hold your breath or overbreathe?

Tension in breathing usually stems from the shoulders. Drop your shoulders and you will breathe more easily. Whenever you are aware of being under stress, breathe out, drop your shoulders, and relax. Your breathing will respond immediately and become rhythmic and even.

When you take time to relax notice how you are breathing. Breathe smoothly and slowly so that it feels as if you are breathing down into your pelvis and touching your baby with your breath. When your breathing is relaxed, your baby will often become active.

Breathing in labour

During labour, these long slow breaths will help at the onset and the end of every contraction. You may be able to breathe like this right through a contraction too. But many women feel the need to breathe more quickly as contractions become more powerful and are closer together. If this is how it is for you, let your breathing speed up and at the same time make it lighter. Rapid deep breathing will result in hyperventilation (see top of page). Rapid light breathing at the height of contractions can help you scale the peaks.

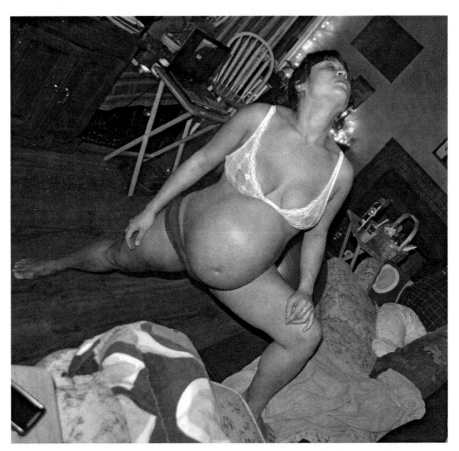

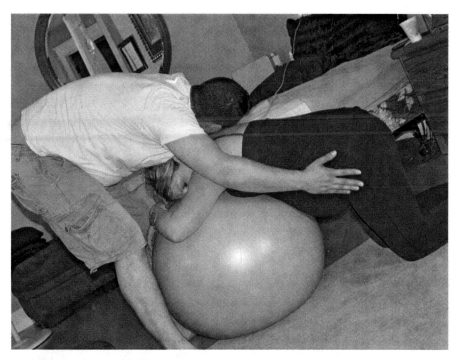

When contractions are at their strongest, it is impossible to move the abdominal wall or to feel anything in your pelvis other than the power of the contractions. The tightening of longitudinal muscle fibres results in a lifting of the abdominal wall, because the contraction causes the top of the uterus, the fundus, to tilt forwards. This swelling also presses against the diaphragm so from your diaphragm down, you will feel as if you are one huge contraction. Let your breathing 'dance' above this and breathe through parted lips with the tip of your tongue resting against your lower teeth. Have sips of water or ice to suck in the spaces between contractions, so that your mouth does not get dry. Avoid huffing and puffing. Your breath should be as light as a whisper. Then, as the contraction reaches its climax and starts to fade, you can form slow, full breaths again. It is important not to forget to do this. You and your baby will welcome the extra oxygen as each contraction finishes. The slow breathing will help you to relax completely in the trough between the great waves of contractions so you are refreshed and strong for the next contraction.

As the contraction reaches its climax and starts to fade, you can form slow, full breaths again

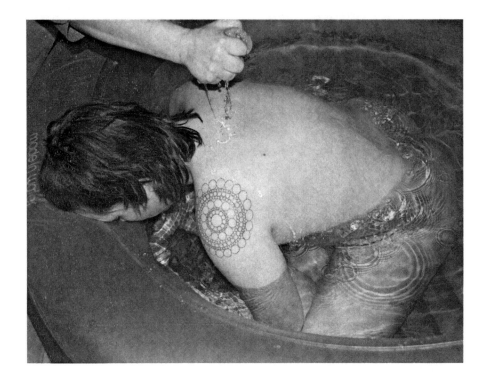

Taught breathing

Breathing is often taught in antenatal classes as a set of exercises, and sometimes these are very rigid and mechanical. It may be that when a woman is giving birth on alien territory, in a hospital where she is not sure what will happen to her, or what she will be allowed to do, such precise techniques are helpful as a distraction from pain and, above all, from an environment that she sees as threatening. The breathing exercises keep her busy and concentrated on something she can do to help herself. I have seen women with their eyes fixed on a crack in the ceiling breathing desperately, as if clinging to a safety rope above a precipice, mentally cut off from their surroundings, unable to hear what anyone is saying, completely out of touch with help that is being offered. When breathing is used like this, it becomes a barrier against the environment.

You will not need to use rigid breathing if you are having your baby at home, or in the kind of out-of-hospital setting where your attendants are already friends, and where there is no need to fear intrusion.

You won't need rigid breathing at home or in a birth centre

Breathing your baby out

When your cervix is wide open and your body ready for the baby to be pushed down, your breathing changes, often dramatically. There is an involuntarily held breath that starts as a catch in the throat. This is a sign that the baby is well on its journey and that you can help it out. While you can continue to breathe, you should do so. Do not attempt to hold your breath deliberately, as this forces the pace and causes unnecessary stress on your pelvic floor muscles and perineum. Then, when you get an irresistible desire to push, drop your jaw, and let yourself open up, and breathe again as soon as the urge passes.

The baby's head will press deeper and deeper until you feel it bulging against your perineum like a grapefruit. You can put your hand down and touch it. From this point on, it is important to breathe your baby out, so that you push only when you cannot resist doing so. Your uterus will do the work for you. Breathing through your open, relaxed mouth, in long sighs, will help your perineum relax and unfold as the baby's head oozes through.

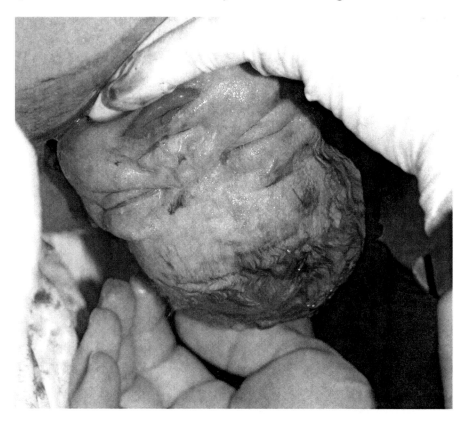

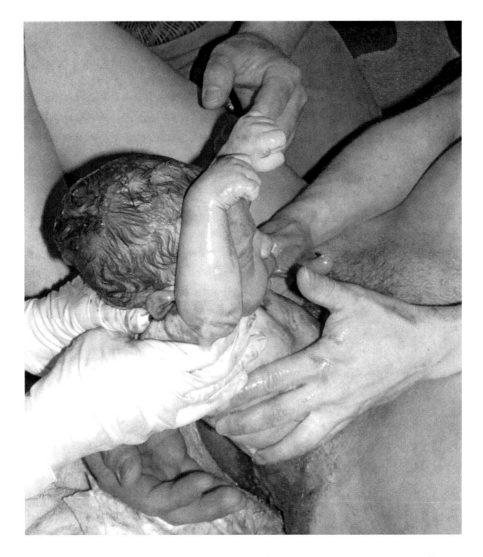

Then the shoulders slide through and, often in one quick movement, like a fish leaping, the whole body emerges, to reveal your slippery, warm, wriggling, wonderful baby. If you are in a pool and the baby is born out of the water it should not be dunked after it is breathing.

Breathing through your open, relaxed mouth will help your perineum relax and unfold as the baby's head oozes through

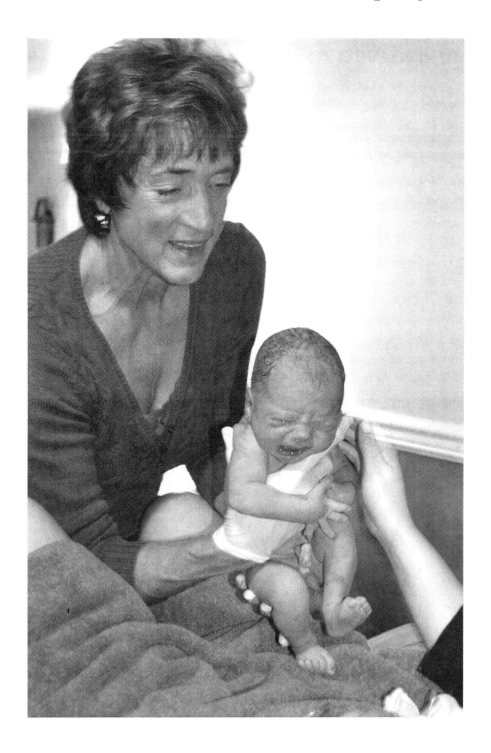

TUNING IN TO YOUR BABY

If you do not wish professional caregivers to take over in childbirth, manage your labour actively and make decisions without consulting you, it is important that you are in touch with your own feelings, with your body and the drama that is unfolding within it, and also with your baby. This little person is carried on the same waves of energy that will sweep through you to the shores of life, and he or she will share the experience with you.

The relationship with your baby starts long before your child is born, long before the very first contractions that herald labour. It has its tentative beginnings as soon as you are aware that you may have conceived, and ripens as you 'listen' to your child's movements and conduct a two-way conversation with the world outside and the one within you. When you are in touch with your baby in the uterus, birth is only one stage in the development of a relationship that is already a reality.

A baby does not suddenly spring into action at birth. For some time before the event your baby has been a complex, coordinated human being who is already learning and communicating.

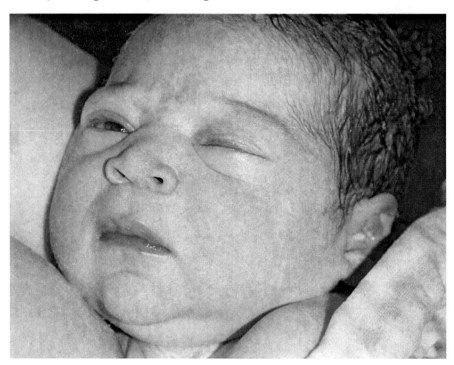

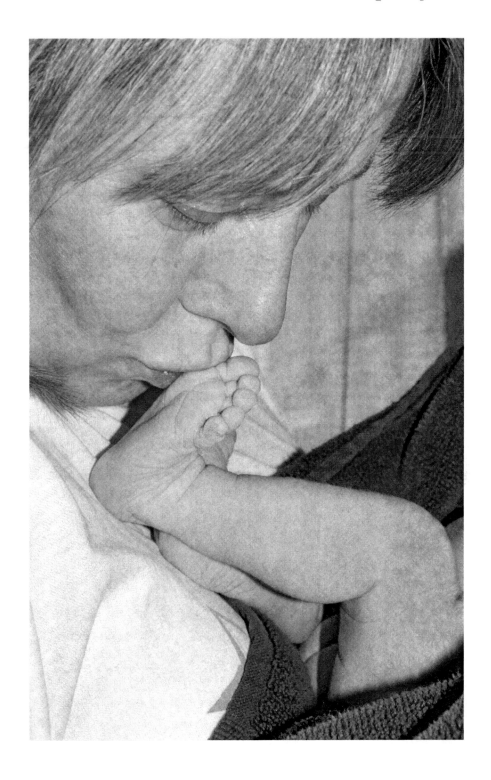

THE POWER OF TOUCH

Babies react to touch very early, although at first this is merely a reflex response. By the time you are 12 weeks' pregnant the baby is already kicking, but you do not feel it at this stage, because he or she is still too small. You usually feel movements for the first time between 17 and 20 weeks. They are like bubbles popping or minnows darting about. But even before that the baby can make complicated foot movements, twisting his or her foot round, curling and uncurling toes, and 'treading water'.

At 16 weeks the baby reaches out with tiny hands, feeling the fluid, exploring the space around and pushing the springy walls of the uterus. Ultrasound reveals that babies often suck their thumbs, so pleasure from non-nutritive sucking is already well-established in the uterus. It assists the coordination of sucking and swallowing necessary for feeding. All the movements that the baby makes have the effect of toning its muscles, in the same way that regular exercise undertaken by adults results in muscular development and strengthening.

66 This child seems to understand laughter or, if we are all shouting and laughing, it starts kicking rhythmically. It touches with its feet anything placed over my abdomen. It feels like delicate exploring. There is an interval during which the baby must be locating the sensation, then a light kick in exactly the right spot.

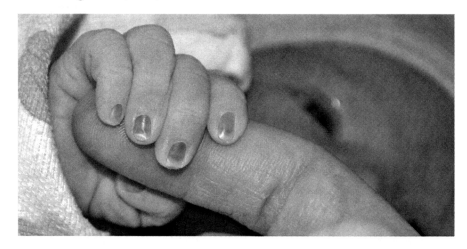

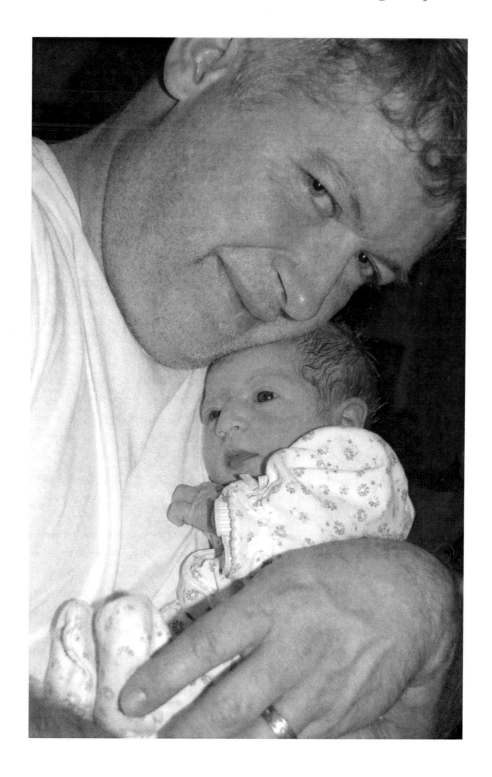

WHAT POSITION IS MY BABY IN?

In the last few weeks of pregnancy you will probably be able to tell the position your baby is in by tracking your baby's legs and trunk with your fingers. When your midwife or doctor palpates your uterus, he or she feels for the head first, but for you it is easier to start with the feet, which may be so clearly defined that you feel you could almost measure the baby for shoes. Starting from where you can find a vigorous little foot, pass your fingers along the legs to the baby's pointed bottom, and then feel down the long curve of the back.

If you are giving birth out of hospital, it will help to know your baby's position

If you are giving birth out of hospital, it will help to know if your baby is head down, if the head is engaged in your pelvis, and whether your baby's back is towards your front with the head tucked forwards on the chest. When this is the case, you can be increasingly confident that the birth will be straightforward.

When your baby is head down (in the vertex or cephalic position), you will feel the kicking in the upper part of the uterus. When your baby's head is up, you will feel the hard ball of the head under your ribs, although you may be deceived by a big baby who is lying head-down with his or her bottom positioned high under your ribs.

Once the head is engaged, your diaphragm can swing down more easily than before as you take a deep breath. When your bladder is full, your baby's head may cause pressure against it so that you want to empty your bladder often, as in the first weeks of pregnancy. This is one sign that the head is deep in the pelvis. Another is an occasional tingling in your vagina. The baby may be using your pelvic floor muscles as a trampoline, giving you short, sharp buzzing sensations like tiny electric shocks. These are signs that the baby is in a very good position.

When the baby is curled into a ball with the back towards your front (in the anterior position), your navel protrudes and you can trace a firm, melon-shaped arc at the front: this is the baby's back. You will also be able to feel kicking at one side or the other under your ribs. Kicking occurs at the side opposite the baby's back.

If your baby is not yet anterior, you will feel kicking all over your front, and there will be a saucer-shaped dip around your navel. This suggests that the baby is posterior, with its back towards your spine. Strong contractions will be needed to turn your baby round into the ideal position for birth. Welcome them when they come and prepare for a long first stage while your uterus does this work. This would mean a backache labour because the hard back of the baby's head would be pressed into the small of your back. Discuss with your caregivers and birth partner how you would handle that.

> If your baby is posterior, welcome any strong contractions because these are needed to turn round a posterior baby

A breech baby

If your baby is still not head down in the last weeks, you can try a pelvic tilt to shift the baby's bottom up out of your pelvis and enable him or her to somersault and turn head down. You will need to get your head lower than your pelvis, either by lying with your pelvis propped up over a couple of firm floor cushions or a beanbag with your head on the floor, or by supporting your pelvis on a low divan bed and leaning over the side of it. Lie turned towards your front rather than your back as the baby will probably find it easier to move against your abdominal wall than against your spine. Make as much space as possible for your baby to move by ensuring that your knees are well apart and not pressing against your abdomen. Now try moving your pelvis to encourage the baby to shift. Rolling and rocking movements are good. This is more likely to be effective at a time when you know the baby is awake and on the move. Although this may not be a posture you would choose for relaxation, once you are reasonably comfortable, relax and give long, slow, full breaths into your pelvis and release your abdominal muscles with each breath out.

Some babies somersault, but then turn back soon afterwards. Others refuse to budge at all. But, if your baby is still breech at the end of pregnancy, it is a manoeuvre worth trying for about 15 minutes, two or three times a day.

> If your baby is breech at the end of pregnancy, the pelvic tilt is a manoeuvre worth trying two or three times a day.

HOW DO I MAKE A BIRTH PLAN?

Discussing your ideas about the birth with whoever is going to attend you in labour helps you focus your mind on what is most important to you and enables your midwife, GP or consultant to understand your needs.

In hospital, birth plans are often presented by anxious women, who are afraid that they will not be consulted about what is done to them during childbirth, to professionals who often feel very threatened by them. I have heard a birth plan described by an obstetrician as 'a weapon used to manipulate the professionals' and by a psychotherapist as 'a transitional object', like a security blanket.

66 "Birth plan?" said the doctor. "What do you want?" I began to explain. "What kind of things do you want to avoid, lovey?" she asked. I said I was not too keen on an episiotomy. She was absorbed in her own calculations. Suddenly she informed me that I was to be admitted straight away, as the baby had not grown in a fortnight. Labour might be induced that very afternoon. So much for my birth plan.

One woman's birth plan:

I would like to:

- ♥ walk around for as long as I like

- ♥ stand or squat during contractions

- ♥ find out for myself the easiest and most comfortable position when pushing

- ♥ have the comforting presence of a close friend who has two children herself

- ♥ have the same midwife present throughout—one who has given me antenatal care, whom I trust and with whom I have a personal relationship

- ♥ have no drugs

  I would like to have the same midwife present throughout

A birth plan helps communication with your caregivers

When you are having your baby out of hospital a birth plan is a valuable element in the communication between you and your caregivers—part of the developing relationship with them. It ought to be like this in hospital too, but often isn't. Another problem with hospital birth plans is that, although you may be encouraged to make a plan, the person with whom you discuss what you want is unlikely to be with you right through labour, so a written birth plan becomes merely a set of orders handed over to a stranger. In the words of one irritated hospital administrator: "It happens in no other branch of medicine or other professional sphere that the client imposes crucial restrictions on the professional and tells him how to do his work." Discussions you have with your caregivers and the decisions to which you come are part of the vital process of getting to know your caregivers, so that by the time you are in labour there is an understanding deeper than words.

Discuss with your midwife, or the small group of midwives who will look after you, the kind of care you would like, whom you want with you during labour, what your partner's role is likely to be, how you would prefer your newborn baby to be treated, and exactly what you are hoping for with this birth. Think about interventions you would prefer to avoid and alternative ways of coping with difficulties. Discuss positions and movements you may want to choose, how you can get physical support for them, whether you want to use a birthing pool, and your thoughts about episiotomy, the clamping and cutting of the umbilical cord, and the conduct of the third stage. Then write down your decisions about the most important issues, if possible on just one sheet of paper. Ask your caregiver how it reads and whether she or he is happy with it. Provide one copy to go with your records and keep another yourself. If by any chance the person you are expecting to attend you in labour is not available, this birth plan will be invaluable and give a clear idea of your preferences.

66 *"Are you going to make a birth plan?" the midwife asked. "I think it's a good idea. We need to discuss ways in which you want to handle pain, so that I can help you. I think our ideas are much the same, but trust between us can't take the place of really knowing what you want."*

HOW CAN I ARRANGE THE ROOM?

You and your partner will want to create your own birth space. This is a kind of 'nesting'. Other mammals and birds line their nests with soft hay or moss, and in most human cultures the mother and those close to her prepare a special room. The Maori birth hut was actually called 'the nesting house' and traditionally, in many parts of North and South America and Asia, women built their own birth huts, often close to water so that they could bathe after the baby was born. The space for receiving the baby was always constructed to be soft and warm. The Kwakiutl of British Columbia used to dig a shallow pit and line it with soft cedar bark, and the Pima of the American South West lined their birth pits with soft rabbit skin. Making one's own birth space is an important part of human culture, which is often neglected nowadays under the assumption that this space is designed to meet the needs of the professionals who conduct the birth, rather than the mother's, and that any personal touches are introduced merely as concessions to her.

Prepare your birth space

Things you may want to get together for an out-of-hospital birth:

♥ beanbags or large floor cushions

♥ a camera

♥ an extra memory card, in case you want to take lots of photos after the birth

♥ sanitary pads, largest size and 'big knickers' to hold them in place

♥ cotton pyjama tops, short nightdresses, or baggy T-shirts

♥ a face cloth

♥ swimwear for your birth partner, so that he or she can go under the shower or into the bath or pool with you if you wish

♥ socks for cold feet

♥ nursing bras

♥ two small real sponges, one to suck on while the other one is in a bowl of cold water

- ♥ a new small plant spray, filled with ice cold water to spray on your face

- ♥ crushed ice to suck

- ♥ MP3 player with your choice of music

- ♥ candles and matches

- ♥ massage and aromatherapy oils (provided you have checked they are safe for use in pregnancy and labour)

- ♥ brush and comb, as well as scrunchies, hairbands or clips to hold long hair away from your face and neck

- ♥ books and/or magazines

- ♥ snacks for your birth partner and midwife

- ♥ honey, glucose drink, or herb teas

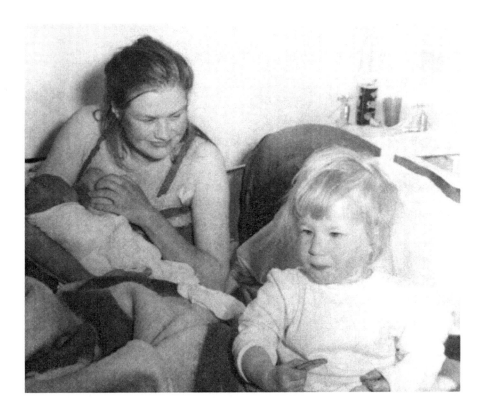

- ♥ bendy straws

- ♥ a rolling pin with a cloth tied over it, or a wooden rolling massager, for back massage

- ♥ paintings, photographs and/or sculptures, to use as a visual focus

- ♥ champagne or another celebration drink and food for after the birth

For birth away from home:

- ♥ a spare can of petrol or diesel, in case you run out of fuel

- ♥ your mobile phone (which needs to have credit on and be charged up)

- ♥ coins or cards for a public phone (in case there is poor reception)

- ♥ a list of telephone numbers

- ♥ baby clothes and clothes you can both wear when you go home

For birth at home—your midwife may provide some of these:

- ♥ two buckets, one for sitting on, one for cleaning up

- ♥ a new nail brush

- ♥ bin liners

- ♥ incontinence pads for sitting on—useful if your waters are leaking or you have a heavy show, as well as for afterwards so that bedding stays clean

- ♥ cleaning cloths

- ♥ a bowl for receiving the placenta

- ♥ a portable lamp

- ♥ some large towels, one for you, one for the baby, one for the midwife

- ♥ a heavy plastic sheet to put over the bed

- ♥ tarpaulin or builders' plastic sheeting to lay over the carpet

If it's cold, get some extra heating, or a fan if it's hot

❝ If you are tired and aching, the first thing you want to do is have a bath. That's why I have hired a birthing pool.

♥ extra heating if it's cold, or a fan if it's hot—or preferably both, in case you or your baby get cold after the birth

♥ frozen peas to act as a cold compress, with a cloth to wrap round the bag of peas, so that you can comfortably rest it against your skin

♥ a small hot water bottle which can be used as a hot compress

♥ a birthing pool—or, if you want to soak in deep water and do not have a birthing pool, plasticine to plug the bath overflow

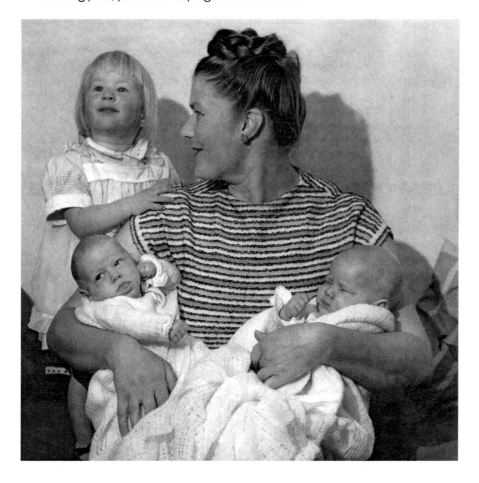

WHAT WILL MY MIDWIFE HAVE WITH HER?

She'll have a delivery pack, which will include the following:

- ♥ a sphygmomanometer to take your blood pressure

- ♥ a Pinard stethoscope and/or a Sonicaid

- ♥ urine-testing sticks

- ♥ local anaesthetic and syringes

- ♥ scissors

- ♥ suturing material, in case of damage to the perineum

- ♥ a mucus extractor, in case the baby's respiratory tract needs clearing

- ♥ resuscitation equipment, in case the baby needs help to breathe

- ♥ an intravenous set and an infusion, in case of bleeding

- ♥ some syntometrine and syringes, in case the uterus needs help to contract to expel the placenta

CREATING COMFORT & THE RIGHT ATMOSPHERE

Have something to help make the room your personal space

If you are going to a birth centre or midwifery-led unit take things with you that will help you or your birth partner(s) make the room your personal space. You could take a painting, some photographs, a plant or a hanging mobile perhaps.

If you are giving birth at home, you may want to choose a room that is small, dark and private. The birthplace does not have to be the bedroom, although a big double bed is lovely if there is room in it for the whole family just after the birth. If you have a garden, you may want to be outside for a time, and squat holding on to a tree when contractions come.

The birthplace does not have to be the bedroom, although a big double bed is lovely if there is room in it for the whole family just after the birth

When you are on dry land, have a stool or beanbag, or a bucket with a rolled towel around the rim, ready to support you in a squatting position. A lunge position with the forward knee bent is easily adopted on the stairs, or with one foot up on a small stool—or on a few large books. The banisters or bathroom towel rail may be the right height to provide a good squatting bar. In rural Africa women often kneel or squat, holding the house post that supports the roof. When my first baby was born, I spontaneously squatted, grasping the heavy, bulbous legs of a Victorian table. It was a hideous table, but good and solid, and felt just right.

With your partner, think what kind of lighting would be best. Lamps that can be dimmed are pleasant. Would you like candles? If your birth attendant wants a bright light on your perineum to see exactly what is happening, how can this be arranged? On a bright day you may like the room flooded with sunlight, or prefer a soft glow through curtains or blinds.

Consider how you will warm and air the room too. You will want to be comfortably warm in labour. In winter you may like to give birth on a hearthrug or a couch in front of the flickering flames of a guarded open fire, or in summer in a room opening onto the garden. You may feel very hot in the second stage and want to have a window wide open or an electric fan available. The baby is emerging from a hothouse atmosphere inside your body, and needs to be born into warm air, so a fan heater that can be switched on as the birth approaches is a good idea.

The baby needs to be born into warm air

USING SOUNDS

Think about the things around you that you will find comforting and that will enhance your positive visualisation of what is happening in your body. If you would like background music, plan this with your birth partner(s). Practise relaxation while this music is playing, so that you associate it with complete release of mind and body. The sounds you choose don't have to be music. You could record the dawn chorus, or waves breaking on the shore. One of my babies was born as a blackbird sang in the apple tree outside my bedroom window. It was an enormously reassuring, happy sound, and I felt that nature was conspiring with me to make the birth beautiful for all of us.

AROMATHERAPY & SMELL

For good smells there is a wide range of aromatherapy oils to choose from. A study of aromatherapy in more than 8,000 births suggests that clary sage and chamomile reduce pain, lavender and frankincense treat anxiety and fear, and peppermint is effective against nausea and vomiting.[11] Be warned, though, that clary sage smells like wet dog... You need to have a head cold or be very fond of dogs! Rose oil is delicious, but expensive, which is the reason why it could not be tested at the Oxford Radcliffe Maternity Hospital. Midwife Ethel Burns introduced aromatherapy there in 1990. One of her aims was to cut the rate of women receiving opiates for pain relief, since pethidine, the most widely used drug, is a very poor analgesic and has side effects for both mother and baby. As a result, this hospital had the lowest rate of pethidine use of all major maternity hospitals in the country. Aromatherapy changes the whole atmosphere of the birth room. It is not only the mother who becomes more relaxed. The people helping her often feel calmer and happier, too. You may like to have scented candles, bunches of lavender or flowers in the room. When my fourth baby was born, my bedroom was full of bowls of hyacinths and I always associate the heady scent of hyacinths with that particular birth.

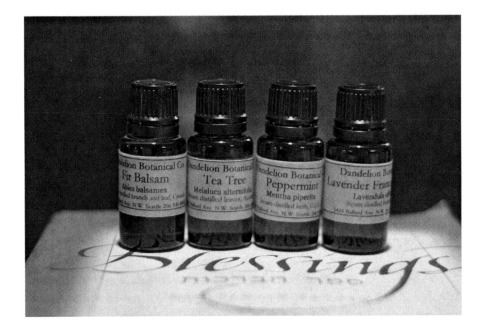

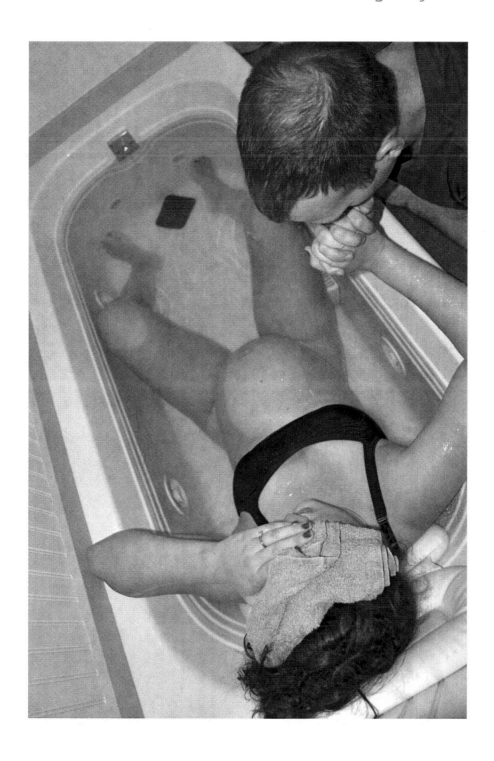

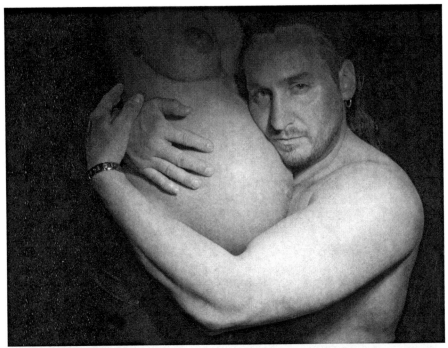

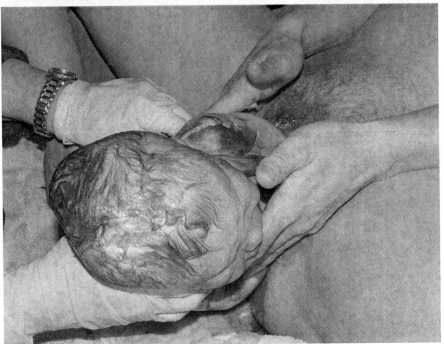

IMAGES OF BIRTH

An important part of your preparation for birth is nothing to do with exercises or information: it is simply to daydream.

An important part of your preparation for birth is nothing to do with exercises or information: it is simply to daydream

When you relax and focus on positive sensory images of birth you open up possibilities for a richer and deeper experience. These images should always be realistic in the sense that they are based on the acknowledgement that labour is stressful, that the power of the uterus is awesome, that when the cervix is opening to its full extent it is usually painful, and that when the baby's head is in your vagina there is an incredible sensation of pressure. You can anticipate and acknowledge all these sensations in a positive way.

THE POWER OF WORDS

The words you use are vital elements in these anticipatory fantasies. Language is never neutral. It presents a view of the world. Most words we have about pregnancy and birth are not only man-made but also medical. A woman is an 'elderly primigravida' or 'high risk'. She has 'an untried pelvis'. Doctors' names are attached to processes in women's bodies as if these medical men had somehow invented them. The contractions in late pregnancy are known as 'Braxton Hicks'. Dilation of the cervix must follow the 'Friedman curve'. (These names are based on the *man* who first wrote about Braxton Hicks in the medical literature and the *man* who first charted the course of some women's labours.)

To use medical language is to impose on yourself a medical view of birth. Sometimes these medical terms are the only words available, so we need to translate them into women's language, and create words that have immediate meaning for us in terms of our own feelings and the ways in which we can express ourselves through our bodies.

Doctors' names are attached to processes in women's bodies as if these medical men had somehow invented them

BODY IMAGES

Your pelvis, for example, is not just an anatomical structure, a piece of architecture through which the fetus is pushed. When you rock your pelvis with your baby nestled inside, it is like a cradle. As you sing, hum or chant, it becomes a resonator. Sometimes it may feel more like a mysterious cave or like a treasure chest that holds the power of the uterus. In a woman's pelvis the ebb and flow of menstrual tides take place and, when the time is right, the full drama of birth is enacted. You can create your own images. You need not use second-hand ones. Here's one I created...

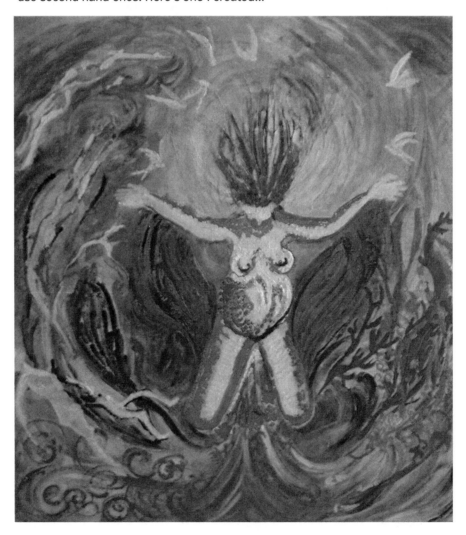

These anticipatory fantasies derived from sensory experience need not all be visual. They can be auditory, for example, based on passages from music and ideas of cadence, harmony, rhythm and being in tune with your body.

They can be tactile too. A feeling of the baby moving inside you is one of intense and often surprising touch. As the uterus contracts and your baby moves down to enter the world, you feel intense pressure, your waters may break with a soft splash, and you are aware of your baby's firm head sliding down—solid and as rounded as a grapefruit—and of quivering, throbbing heat as the head crowns. As it slips forwards and you reach down to feel it, your fingers touch soft, wet hair, and you are astonished at the otherness of this little creature who has for so long been a part of yourself but is now being born from your body.

Kinetic images may come to mind too. Your breathing dances, you get into the swing of contractions, swimming over each as it rises in crescendo, or breasting it like a great ocean wave. You float, you ride, you ski down the mountain slopes, you leap into the void. I shall never forget an Israeli woman who, as each contraction swelled up, proclaimed: "Gates of Jerusalem, open for me!" And for her this was the intense image that most accurately expressed the sense of her body opening wide as she gave birth.

Imagery likely to be helpful will include active verbs of opening, releasing, spreading, unfolding and fanning out

The imagery that is likely to be helpful to you will include active verbs of opening, releasing, spreading, unfolding, and fanning out. As contractions sweep through you, concepts that suggest power, energy, strength and, perhaps, storm and even whirlwind suddenly make sense, along with wave and water fantasies—verbs such as stream, pool, flood, gush, flow and cascade may come to mind. And all over the world, in many different cultures, women use visual images of fruit ripening and of the baby's head like a hard bud in the centre of a flower's unfurling petals.

As you read about birth, and whenever you take time to relax and enjoy anticipatory fantasies, create your own images and dreams that will give positive meaning to all the sensations of labour. Doing this will help you savour fully an adventure that can be among the most thrilling, intense and satisfying experiences of your life.

WATER BIRTH

You may want to use water—in a bath, shower, jacuzzi, or a special birthing pool. If so, do you want your partner to be in the water with you or not? You may feel differently when you are in labour, but plan ahead for a range of possibilities and experiment with different positions and movements in water.

> You may feel differently when you are in labour, but plan ahead for a range of possibilities and experiment with different positions and movements in water

Of course you are concerned about safety. A paediatric study of over 4,000 births in water in the UK between 1994 and 1996 compared with more conventional births to women not at any special risk, showed that water birth is not dangerous. It is as safe for the baby to be born in water as in air.[12]

Labouring in water

It can be easier to relax, move freely and—in the old Quaker phrase—'centre down' in warm water than on dry land. Labouring in water helps create harmony between mind and body and stimulates the spontaneous flow of hormones that enable the uterus to contract, the cervix to open, and the baby to be pressed through bone, muscles and overlapping layers of soft tissue for birth. Randomised controlled trials show that women who labour in water experience less pain and adapt more readily than those on dry land.[13]

There are a variety of birthing pools available for hire to use at home or to take into hospital.

> There are a variety of birthing pools available for hire to use at home or to take into hospital

A parliamentary report (House of Commons Select Committee, 2003) emphasised the key recommendation of two earlier Department of Health publications (1991 and 1993) that all maternity units offer the option of a birthing pool. These pools are usually plumbed in. They cannot be booked in advance and their use may be restricted to women classified as 'low risk'. So it is wise to check this out at an antenatal clinic visit.

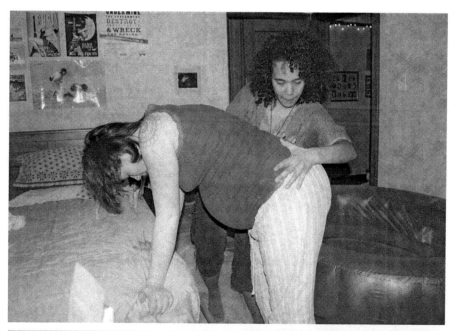

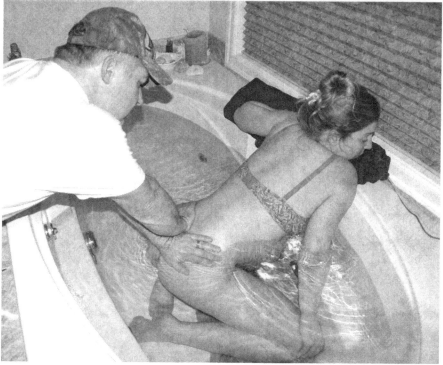

Water birth Q&A:

Q: Where shall we set up the pool?

A: The ideal room for a birthing pool is probably on the ground floor, with one door opening out onto a garden and another onto a darkened, comfortable room where you can escape the pressures of the outside world and sink deeply into your own sensations. If it is warm weather, you can labour part of the time in the fresh air, then withdraw to your womb-like room or float peacefully in the pool the rest of the time. The important thing is to be free to move between these environments and not feel committed to water birth, come what may.

The ideal room for a birthing pool is probably on the ground floor, with one door opening out onto a garden and another onto a darkened, comfortable room

Q: Are the floor boards strong enough?

A: If you want to have the pool in an upstairs room and the floor is wooden, check with the people from whom you are hiring it or a friendly builder that the floor can take its weight when it is filled with water. The filled pool will weigh about one tonne.

Q: Can the hosepipe reach the taps?

A: There are two hoses with the pool. One has attachments to connect it securely to the taps. Allow a good hour to fill the pool. The second enables you to run off water, so that you can feed in fresh hot water through the other hose or empty the pool. To avoid having hosepipes snaking all over the place, the pool is best located not far from a sink or bath. Can the pool be emptied easily? Think about where the waste water will run—perhaps straight into a drain or garden. A pool equipped with an electric pump can be emptied rapidly.

If you want to have the pool upstairs and the floor is wooden, check the floor can take its weight when filled with water

Q: How do we heat the water?

A: It helps to have an efficient domestic hot water supply. If necessary, turn up the thermostat on the immersion heater, but be very careful if you have other children in the house. Some pools have heaters similar to those used in aquaria. Although they maintain the water at a constant temperature, they are not powerful enough to heat it from cold, and you may not like the idea of having a heater in the pool when you are in it. The pool should have a plastic cover that retains heat well, even without a heater, so that once filled it will stay warm for eight to 10 hours.

Q: What temperature should the water be?

A: Around blood temperature is right. Really hot water is not good for the baby, who—while inside you—is hotter than you. The air around the pool should be warm so that after the birth the baby does not lose heat rapidly and so that you can cuddle her while still sitting in the water. In the second stage you may get very hot, and it will feel good if the water is cool. This will help you mobilise your energy to push the baby out and will stimulate the urge to bear down.

Q: When should we get the pool?

A: Set the pool up about 10 days before the baby is due and use it for relaxation and centring down into positive thoughts about the birth. It helps to alleviate late-pregnancy backache and feels good if you have clusters of painful Braxton Hicks contractions or a long lead-in to labour.

Q: How can the water be kept clean?

A: Empty the pool every 24 hours or so and refill with clean water. It is usually not difficult to keep the water clean. A plastic sieve can be used to scoop any debris out of the water.

Q: Is it safe to leave the baby underwater after the birth?

A: No. At birth, gently lift your baby's head free of the water. Don't jerk it up suddenly—this may cause a short cord to break. Although this is not an emergency and a midwife knows what to do, it is best avoided and the cord can be left intact to stop pulsating by itself.

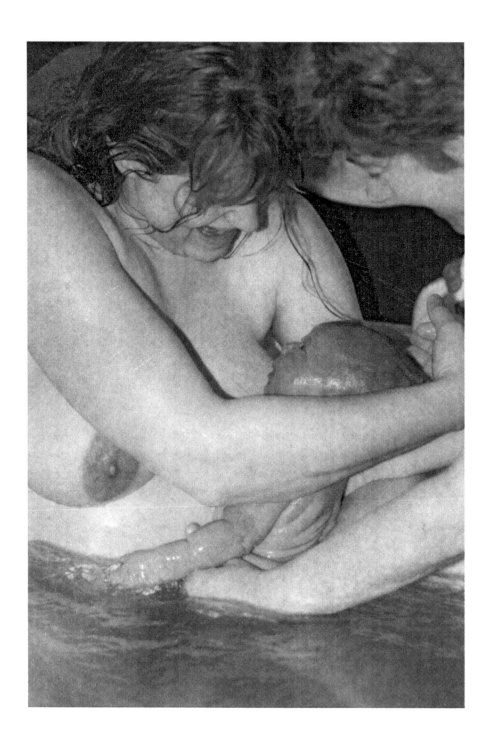

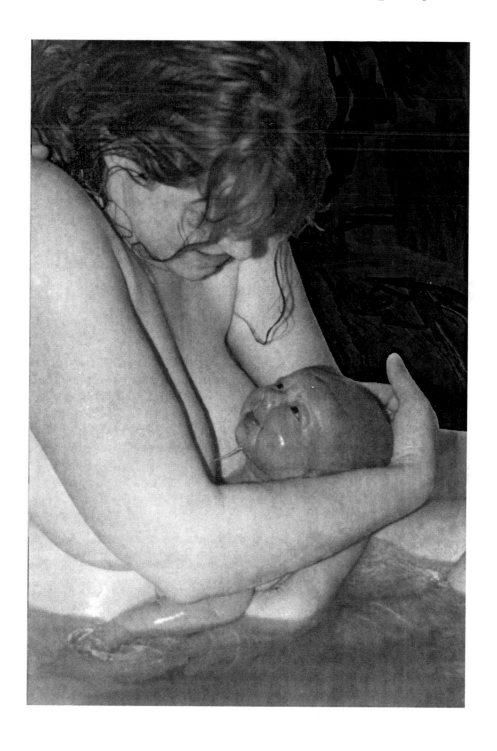

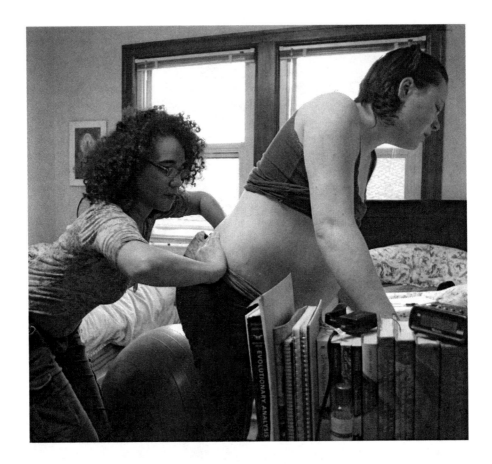

Your birth partner

Sharing the experience of childbirth with someone who is close to you helps give you strength and confidence. When you have a baby at home this person is usually your sexual partner because birth occurs quite naturally as part of the flow of your relationship. When birth is in a birth centre or midwifery-led unit, you may want your sexual partner with you as this special person, or you may want someone else—an intimate friend or relative.

MALE ANXIETIES ABOUT BIRTH

66 Chris was looking at the baby with his complete attention, his face transfigured with happiness and wonder. He looked like a small child seeing something more wonderful than he had ever seen before.

In the past men distanced themselves from birth, both its physiological and emotional aspects. It was not 'manly' to do anything else. They strode the hospital corridors while their wives laboured. They crouched, smoking in the fathers' waiting room. They went to a pub and drank themselves silly to anaesthetise their fears. Or they tried to concentrate on work as if nothing important was happening. They denied the strength of their own anxiety. It was as if a script was already written for them and they had to accept their allotted roles. Men lost out as well as women. The taboo on tenderness, of which this was one example, meant that they were expected to be strong to shoulder burdens, to earn money to support their wives and children, and to protect territory, but were not allowed to be aware of the intricacies of human emotion or the subtleties of relationships. If they were, they had to put on an act and pretend that they were tough and strong. The role stereotype was basically ape-like, not human.

In the span of 50 years, fathers' involvement in childbirth in Western culture, novel in the 1960s, has come to be accepted

In the span of 50 years, fathers' involvement in childbirth in Western culture, novel in the 1960s, has come to be accepted as normal. Maybe the idea of fathers at birth contained the seed of 'the new man'—the male personality who is not grabbing, fighting and crude, but who can be nurturing and tender. But in spite of attending the births of their babies, this new man is a much heralded but still rare creature—a new and endangered species in a rough, tough world. Yet each time a woman gives birth and a man has the opportunity to share the experience and to grow in understanding, there is at least a chance that not only a baby will be born, but also a man with a deeper awareness and sensitivity.

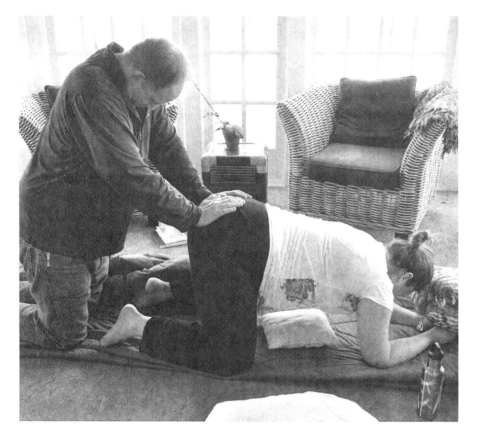

On the other hand it is easy to be over-optimistic about the changes that can be brought about when fathers are involved in childbirth in hospital. A concerned, caring father can help with communication and give his partner strong emotional support. But hospitals are organised so that even the most determined man may go along with the system all too easily and fail to give the support a woman needs.

When fathers began to be at births back in the 1960s, their presence was at first resisted by many doctors and midwives, who felt that their territory was threatened. But within a few years fathers came to be warmly welcomed, as staff realised that most of them turned into subordinate, well-behaved members of the birth 'team', who could be relied upon to help control the woman's behaviour, keep her calm, and make her 'see reason' when staff wished to intervene against her wishes.[1]

Men still often feel out of place in hospital childbirth, and do everything they can to maintain good relations with staff, to be polite and compliant, and to prevent the woman 'making a fuss' or drawing attention to herself. They go into hospital with the firm purpose of giving labour support, but many are cowed into submission by the whole atmosphere and by the evident authority of the senior men (or women) who are in charge. Fathers often feel violent emotions welling up inside them because of how their partners are being treated, yet are conditioned by their education to block the expression of disturbing feelings, and to be obedient team members. In this state of mind they are inclined to play the hospital game, to collude with the medical system, and women are left feeling isolated and abandoned.

Most obstetricians are men, and it is unlikely that this has occurred by chance. They want to control women in the most essentially female activity of giving birth. So they invent machinery to enable them to do this more effectively. It is almost a truism to say that men like machines, enjoy tinkering with them, and rely on them more than women. (It is only a truism, because it is usually women who operate and understand the idiosyncrasies of electric irons and kettles, vacuum cleaners, washing machines, dishwashers, mixers, sewing machines and even home computers.) Because men are accustomed to being in control of women, obstetricians manage childbirth—or at least achieve a semblance of management—with electronic equipment. Prospective fathers are often reassured when they see the technology available in the modern hospital, whereas their female partners tend to be disturbed by it. Of course there are some men who are made equally anxious by all this high-tech gear, just as there are women who breathe a sigh of relief and believe that nothing can go wrong if it is to hand. But they are probably in the minority.

Fathers' sharing in the birth experience can be the stimulus for men's freedom to nurture and a sign of changing relationships between men and women. In the same way, women's freedom to give birth at home is a political decision, an assertion of our determination to reclaim the experience of birth. Birth at home is about changing society.

❝❝ We felt strongly that our child should emerge into her father's arms and share that first breath of life in the intimate bond of the family.

THE DEEPER MEANINGS OF BIRTH

" Nicholas was where I needed him about ten seconds before I knew where that was! I felt supported, but not pushed, by all three of them.

" Philip fixed me with his eyes gently and kindly, yet insistently. He never allowed me to sink into the pain. Eye contact and simultaneous breathing with him got me through the contractions.

A father

" The birth was made much easier by being in comfortable, familiar and planned surroundings, and having midwives who were our friends, rather than the staff of an institution, visiting our own home and helping us through a difficult but exciting and joyful time.

Sharing the experience of birth can be a peak event in a loving relationship, something that is never forgotten. Rahima Baldwin, who helps run a birth centre where half the parents are Arab, speaks movingly of "the profound moment when the father whispers the *al-adhan*, or call to prayer" to his newborn child. Men who were not at all sure at first that they wanted to be present say afterwards: "I wouldn't have missed it for the world." For many it is as if suddenly they are face to face with life's real meaning and a power even more overwhelming than sexual desire.

When women are asked afterwards what their partners did that helped, they often say: "It was just that he was there." Being present in the moment, not distracting or distracted, but right there with the woman, is the essence of being a birth partner. It is nothing to do with coaching the woman, as the father's role is often described in North American childbirth education. It is not a matter of complicated techniques, but of giving her complete and focused concentration.

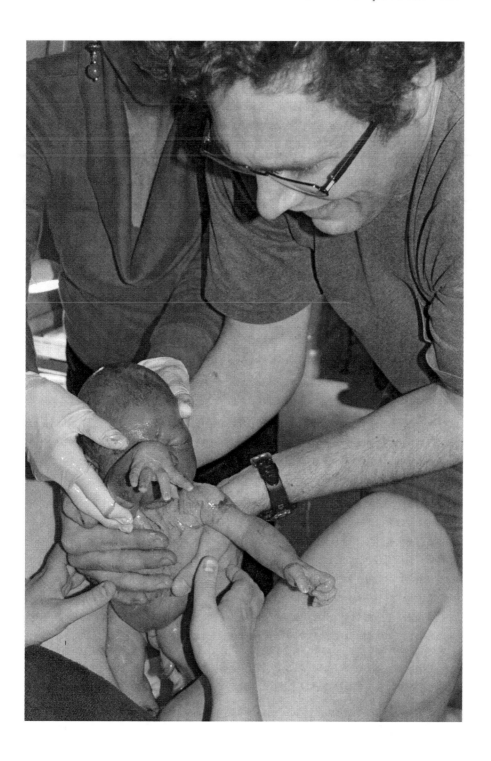

It is possible to be physically present with a woman in labour and not be there at all

It is possible to be physically present with a woman in labour and not be there at all. I remember accompanying one couple having a hospital birth for whom the event was a truce in a long, drawn-out battle. The husband, who was a doctor, brought his radio into the delivery room and, as his wife was pushing the baby out, he switched on the news and listened to it intently, until I suggested that this was the wrong time and place for it and asked him to get behind her to support her head and shoulders. It may be that delivery rooms and women in the second stage were so commonplace for him that he did not see any need to be emotionally involved. Or he may have been trying to punish his wife. Or perhaps he was trying to protect himself from overwhelming emotion and was frightened that he might feel too much.

PREPARING TOGETHER

Your birth partner can prepare with you for the birth, not just be called in when you start labour. He or she should be someone who understands your needs and knows exactly when it is appropriate to give help and when to stand back.

Men are often poorly prepared for the experience of childbirth. A study of what fathers actually did when they had planned to act as 'labour coaches' in a Canadian hospital revealed that they spent a lot of time trying to hide their feelings and worrying that they were not being useful.[2]

Although most had attended childbirth classes, they were not able to help in the way they had expected, and their emotions proved very different from those anticipated. Since the hospital environment often inhibits a man from giving his partner full support it puts him under great stress. He feels surrounded by experts, is scared of doing the wrong thing and, if the woman becomes distressed as labour progresses, he becomes increasingly anxious. Birth in an out-of-hospital setting provides an environment in which the birth partner can also be himself. He doesn't feel that he has to put on an act.

In one study most men were not able to help in the way they had expected and their emotions were not as anticipated

Sharing your feelings about birth

Anyone who is present at a birth brings to it their own emotions, their own expectations, their fear and hope, and their love. As a baby is born, there is not only the mother's birth passion, but the often intense emotions of all others involved. This is why emotional preparation is vital. Childbirth education is not just a matter of learning what happens and knowing how to help. It should be a process that leads to greater self-awareness. Whether your birth partner is your sexual partner or some other person, it is important to talk together about your feelings beforehand. When you do this, consider the following questions together:

♥ What is most important to you about the birth?

♥ What do you want of your birth partner?

♥ How does your birth partner feel about this?

♥ What kind of help will your partner need to give?

♥ How does your partner feel about this?

Emotions about birth are often complex and powerful. You can explore feelings further by each going on to finish the statement, "When I think about the birth, I feel..." Listen to each other without judgement and if some of your emotions turn out to be threatening, do not try to change them or protest that there is no need to feel like this. Just accept them.

> Listen to each other without judgement and if some of your emotions turn out to be threatening, do not try to change them or protest that there is no need to feel like that

Can you remember your first contact with birth as a child? As I talk with couples, I find that earliest memories are often negative. Adults may recall bewilderment and pain when their mother was whisked off to hospital, they were left without her and then presented with a baby who replaced them. They may also remember hushed, pitying voices as 'female problems' were discussed, or an aunt's 'bad time', as women talked in shocked whispers about the number of stitches she had. All these experiences must colour our view of birth, even if only to make us determined to do things differently.

Many men are not sure that they can handle seeing the woman they love in pain, or cope with being close to the sheer physicality of birth. If you have seen a birth film, talk about your feelings as you watched it, too. But when you do so remember that viewing a film is very different from being fully involved in a birth. With a film you are merely a spectator, and there is nothing you can do about it. In a birth you are needed and caught up in the yearning and excitement. It is the difference between watching a film of surfers on Bondi beach in Australia and actually being there and riding the waves yourself.

Talking about how your partner has felt in the past when you have been in pain or were ill or especially vulnerable can also help deepen your understanding of each other. What did you want then? What did he do and was that the right thing for you? When a woman feels trapped and unable to control what other people do to her pain in childbirth is turned into *suffering*. If, on the other hand her birth partners do what she wants them to do, she should be able to remember that the pain of birth is functional, creative, positive—that it is pain with a purpose.

In an intimate atmosphere where there is mutual understanding the physicality of birth can be close to that of lovemaking. The swelling uterus straining against the abdominal wall, the woman's quickened breathing, her damp skin and hair and shining eyes, the astonishing urge to push, the energy that pours through her, the grunts and moans as she presses the baby down, the bulging perineum, the top of the baby's head like a wrinkled walnut in her vagina, then the head oozing through—all these elements in birth are sexual when they are not made medical in the context of hospital care.

Sharing your birth dreams

Women often dream more during pregnancy. Dreams that were previously grey turn technicoloured. Men may dream too, and their dreams may express hopes and anxieties about birth. Sometimes there is fear of losing the woman, the baby being abnormal, or of not being able to measure up to what is required of them. While I am not suggesting that you go into lengthy dream analysis, dreams can often provide clues to the problems we are trying to sort out in our lives and the challenges we face. It helps just to realise this and to say, "Yes, I am worried about it," and think whether there is some positive action that you can take to deal with the challenge. Even when there is nothing practical to be done, simple acknowledgement of fear often enables you to handle it.

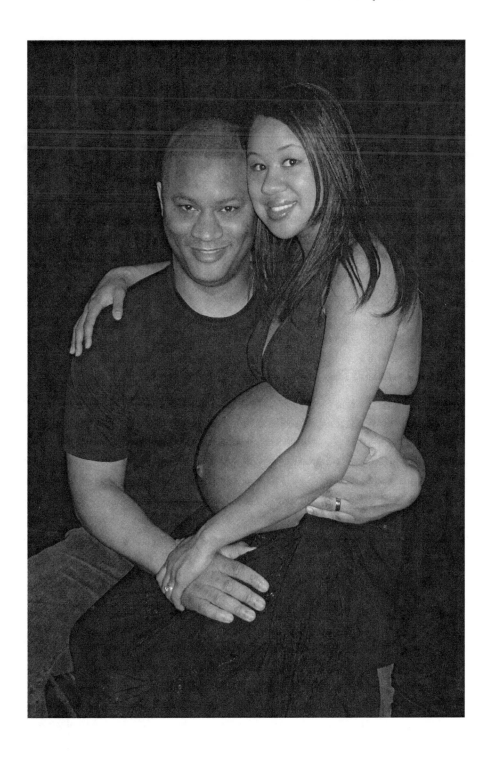

WHAT IF I HAVE A FEMALE FRIEND TO HELP ME?

Sometimes a man wants to be present but feels that he cannot take entire responsibility for giving emotional support. Then, having another person as well, a woman friend who understands birth, may be a good idea. This person may be called a *doula*, a Greek word meaning 'the woman who serves' and, in France, a *monitrice*, which means 'the woman who watches and is aware'. When a couple are together, the task for the doula is not to take over, but to provide support. As one doula put it: "I am there to help a woman, just like her mother or father was when she learnt to ride a bicycle. During birth I am like the parent who held on to the back of the bicycle until the rider had some experience and felt safe and turned around to see that she had been riding on her own for quite some time."[3]

Sometimes a man wants to be present but feels that he cannot take entire responsibility for giving emotional support

CHOOSING THE RIGHT BIRTH PARTNERS

The notion that a woman can have only one companion with her, and that this must be the baby's father, stems from the time in the late 1960s when fathers were first allowed in delivery rooms, and women were told that no one else could possibly come because there was no room. Over and over again senior midwives and doctors explained to couples: "There just isn't space." Notices were often put up by delivery suite doors: "No admission. Fathers only." This was hard on single mothers and on any woman who wanted a woman friend or lesbian partner with her instead of a man.

Now in many countries the father's presence is unquestioned. But in ritualising the attendance of fathers and making it almost mandatory, women are denied the right to choose another person, or perhaps several people with different qualities to offer. It is only in a home setting that these decisions can be made freely; and it is important that they are made, and that a reluctant or anxious father does not hang around simply because he lives there and everyone assumes that he is the obvious birth partner.

In making the attendance of fathers almost mandatory, women are denied the right to choose another person, or several others

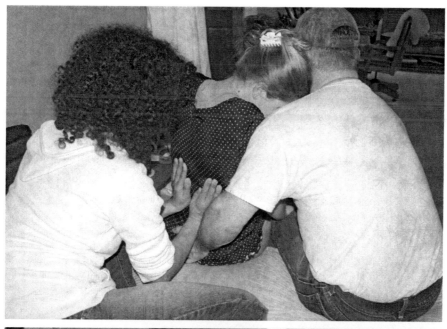

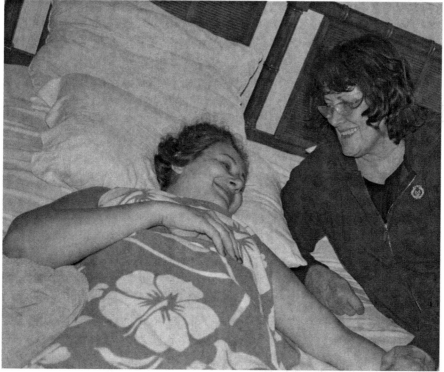

I'M THE BIRTH PARTNER... WHAT DO I DO?!

For the woman you are supporting, you are an anchor in a stormy sea. Being able to remain calmly confident during labour is the single most important quality you need. There are many ways of giving comfort when the going gets tough and of refreshing the woman if she feels so tired that she wishes it was all over. You will learn about these skills in antenatal classes and have a chance to rehearse them and find out what are likely to suit her best. When you do rehearse in a group with other couples, you can learn a great deal from each other and can also share ideas.

It often helps to use words and phrases that were used in the antenatal classes—those that held most meaning for you. They can be very simple—such as "Open", "Release", "Lovely", or "Good"... or repeated phrases, such as "Let it flow", "You're strong", "You're doing really well", "That's another one gone", or "We're getting there." However, using these words and phrases must be done with discretion. No one wants to be hectored or cajoled in labour. If you offer help without empathy it can seem to the labouring woman as if you're taking over, and she may think: "Who's having this baby—you or me?" So keep words to a minimum.

I have found myself in the role of birth partner in countries where I have been studying women's experiences of birth and have not spoken the language. All I needed to do was know a few words, such as "Softly", "Breathe", "Gently", "Open wide", and "Beautiful", with which to reach out to a woman, and these have been enough to give strong birth support. I aim to be beside a woman, not *over* her but *with* her. Separated by culture, education, and language, we still encounter each other as sisters.

Whatever techniques birth partners acquire, however much they learn, the essence of what they give to the woman in birth is that they are her lovers and friends, not assistants to the midwife, barefoot doctors, or labour 'coaches'.

❝I didn't need him to do anything. I didn't want to be told what to do. Being able to rely on him, knowing he wouldn't leave me, seeing him there smiling as I came out of every contraction, that was what I needed.

66 When I was in transition I said "I'm bloody well not doing this again," and he reminded me: "You must be nearly fully dilated. It won't be long now! Take one contraction at a time." When I did that, the pain was suddenly manageable.

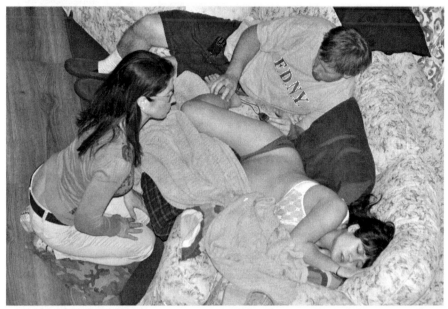

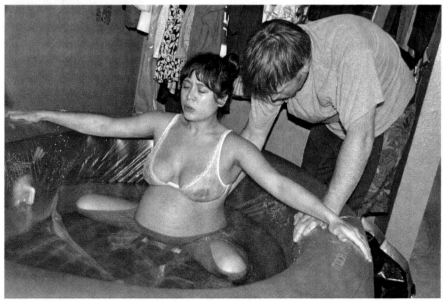

HOW DO I USE TOUCH, MASSAGE & HOLDING?

When a woman feels tossed and lost and broken by fierce contractions coming in quick succession, being held firmly helps her feel safe. Your hand stroking lightly or massaging her deeply can relieve pain even when it is very threatening, depending on where and how the touch is given. Any kind of physical contact from a person whom she trusts can, if given with discretion and sensitivity, help her relax in a situation which is stressful. One strong benefit of not being in an alien environment during labour is that you are much less likely to feel inhibited in giving her physical support and caring for her freely through touch.

During pregnancy you can explore together ways of touching and holding, so that just a look or gesture will indicate to you when and where she wants to feel the reassurance and energy that is given by a loved hand. Before you practise together, you can prepare some massage oil—vegetable oil or nut oil lightly scented with any essential oil that she finds relaxing. Then she strips down to her underclothes and settles in a warm, comfortable place, well supported by pillows. Overleaf are some more suggestions for you.

66 It was good having him to squeeze tight, and I knew he wouldn't mind how hard I squeezed. With anyone else I would have felt bound to apologise, but I just clung on to him.

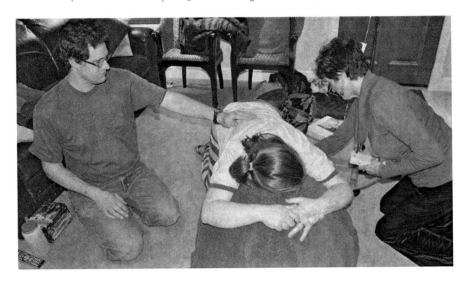

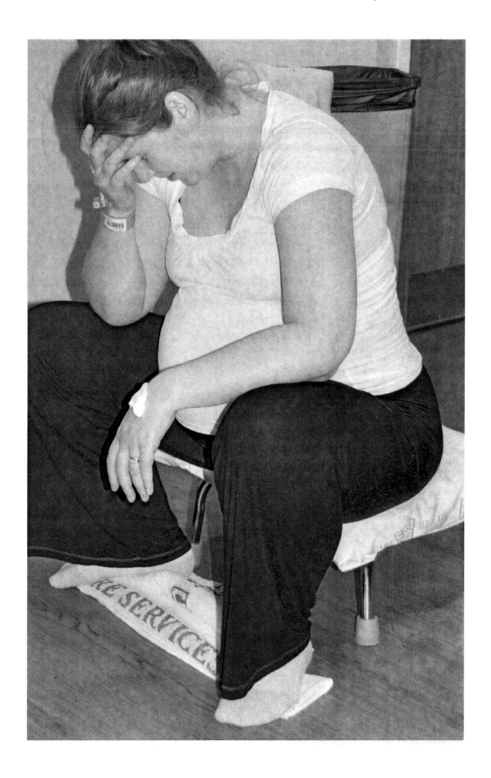

Stroking

You can make contact with the baby by stroking the woman's abdomen lightly. This touch needs to be made with really relaxed, warm hands, so it is worth spending a few minutes loosening your hands before starting by shaking them vigorously from the wrists, as if flicking water from the fingertips. For all massage, your shoulders need to be loose too. If they are tight, tension is conveyed down the arm into the hand and can even cause pain.

Slow, light stroking over the lower abdomen can feel good in labour, especially before 5cm dilation of the cervix. If you are slightly to one side of the woman, an oiled hand can be drawn from underneath the far curve of her abdomen in an arc down over the place where her cervix is dilating and then up again over the nearer side, followed by the other hand using a similar smooth movement in the same direction. The resulting light fingertip massage seems to be stroking the baby's head.

Shoulder massage

The tension that results in overbreathing and hyperventilation starts in the shoulders, and a shoulder massage helps her loosen these muscles. Position yourself behind her, fingers resting on her shoulders, and massage firmly with thumbs in the valleys either side of her spine. Then try moving your thumbs slowly and firmly in a circular motion over her shoulder blades.

66 When contractions are coming every two or three minutes a woman often feels that she needs an anchor in the stormy sea of labour, and wants to be upright and firmly held.

66 My midwife was warm, loving, and calm. She massaged my feet and kept encouraging me. I looked into Nick's eyes and saw the love he has for me. This kept me going through a 36-hour labour.

Long, slow, sweeping movements can help the woman relax

Back massage

Long, slow, sweeping movements with the hands down either side of the labouring woman's spine can help her relax completely between contractions, so that she does not carry tension from one contraction over to another. First rest your hands on her shoulders. Then sweep one hand firmly, but slowly, down her back. When this hand reaches her bottom, let the other hand join in the movement and slowly sweep down the other side, as you replace your first hand on her shoulder, and so on. You will need to have a relaxed body to do this easily as this massage is only satisfying when you literally get into the rhythmic swing of it.

When the woman is experiencing back pain it is usually most concentrated at the sacrum, the big bone where her pelvis is attached to her spine, or to one side of this. Pain in this region is helped by very firm circular massage from the heel of the palm with the other hand resting over it, so that pressure comes from the weight of your back down your shoulders and arms into your hands. When you practise this, try the effect of being at different angles to the woman's body, because the pressure the woman feels will be different depending on whether it is exerted in an upward or downward direction. It may be most effective when you are near her shoulders, so that this pressure is exerted downwards on her sacro-lumbar ligaments.

Foot massage

Hold the woman's feet in your lap and between strong contractions first squeeze her foot above and below her calf muscles front and back, and then massage the soles of her feet with your thumbs. As the next contraction builds up, stop moving your hands and exert firm thumb pressure just below the big toe of each foot, slightly in towards the next toe. If you experiment with this before the woman goes into labour, you will find a spot in which strong pressure produces a slight buzzing sensation. This means you have found an acupressure (shiatsu) pain prevention point.

Giving counterpressure

She may appreciate firm counterpressure rather than moving touch. So much is happening inside her that any movement may be distracting and break her concentration. Counterpressure is particularly effective for low back pain if you rest your hands one on top of the other over exactly the right spot and let your weight flow down your arms. As the baby presses lower she may like this pressure over her buttocks.

Kneading

Deep massage into the flesh and underlying muscles can help her cope with sensations which might otherwise seem preposterous and threatening. As the baby's head presses against her rectum and anus, she may feel as if she is about to empty her bowels. Then, as the head fans out all the tissues, it feels like a huge ball just behind her anus. To help her relax her buttock and pelvic floor muscles, you can knead her buttocks using thumbs or thumbs and fingers, as if kneading bread dough.

Holding

Holding is helpful not only for physical support in upright positions, but when she just needs to know that someone is there, focused entirely on her, or when she wants to be steadied and anchored. Some good holding positions with which you can experiment are: supporting the back of her shoulders; encircling a wrist; grasping her feet; holding the bony ridge of her pelvis on either side; and cradling her head with a hand on each side or one hand cupped over the back of her head. Stay quite still, feeling and sharing the power that is sweeping through her body.

Note: You can find much more about touch, massage, and holding in my book *Pregnancy and Childbirth: Choices and Challenges*.[4]

Deep massage into the flesh and underlying muscles can help the woman cope with sensations which might otherwise seem preposterous and threatening

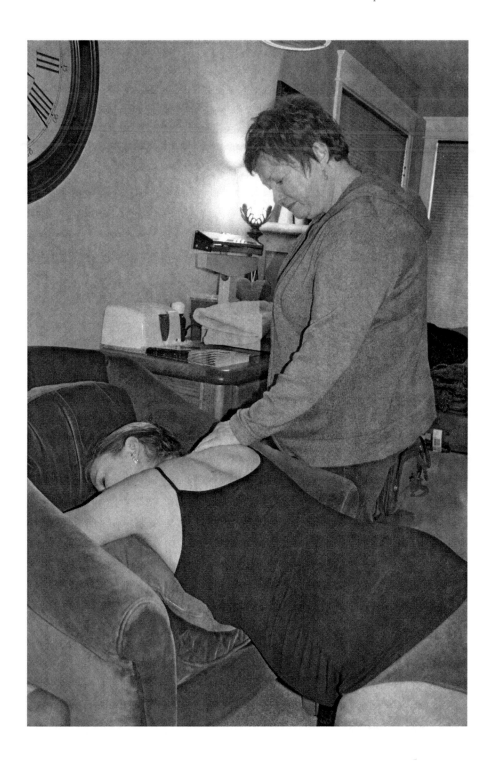

Moving around

When a woman is in labour it will help if she has already explored with you movements and positions she is most likely to find comfortable, bearing in mind as she does so that upright positions will enable her uterus to contract freely and the baby's head to rotate and descend. One great advantage of home birth is that you both already know exactly what you can use for comfort and physical support—walls, window ledges and furniture—and you don't have to use any special apparatus such as a squatting bar or birth chair. Experiment with the following movements and positions together:

♥ While the woman is walking around she can imagine a contraction, then lean back or forward on to you with her legs well apart and knees unlocked. She can try this facing you, behind you, and at your side. Experiment with you standing with your back against the wall for support. Then try it sitting on a chair or table. Find out in which of these positions you have just practised you can rub her back easily. The woman then walks around again and this time imagines contractions with low backache. Try massaging her firmly in the small of her back where her pelvis joins her spine. (Note that massage is best done at one side or both sides of the spine, not right on it, using the heel of the palm rather than the fingers or flat of the hand.)

♥ She walks again and when an imaginary contraction starts, she leans back or forward on to a wall in any way that is comfortable. Massage her as she stands in this position. Continue to massage her as she stands in this position.

♥ She sits facing the back of an upright chair, leaning over a pillow on the back of the chair, with her shoulders rounded, feet flat on the floor. Try massaging her back in this position.

♥ Now she turns so that she is sitting on the chair in the conventional way. Kneel in front of her and let her lean over you.

Upright positions will help the woman's uterus contract freely

There are many other positions and movements you can explore in which you provide support or massage, or sometimes both at once. Sometimes it may feel best to move with the woman, and at other times it will feel more appropriate to remain still. In some or all of the following positions the labouring woman may also welcome additional physical support from you:

♥ when she is kneeling and holding her body upright or alternatively leaning over you, while you are on all fours in front of her

♥ when she is kneeling, her legs apart, leaning forward, with her head on a pillow on a chair in front of her

♥ when she is half-kneeling, half-squatting, with one foot on the floor

♥ when she is squatting, leaning forward with her hands on the floor

♥ when she is in an all-fours position, perhaps rocking her pelvis with you resting a hand at either side of her pelvis

♥ when she is squatting, leaning forward (holding on to you) and then rocking her pelvis to and fro

In the peace between contractions you may like to use some of the following phrases or questions so that the woman can be your guide:

♥ Do you want to be touched or not?

♥ Would you like me to move my hands, or keep them still?

♥ Will you guide my hands?

♥ Heavier? Lighter?

♥ Shall I talk you through the next contraction, or be quiet?

♥ Show me how to hold you.

♥ Does it help if I breathe with you?

Don't say these things all at once. Use your words with discretion. The woman in labour leads. You follow.

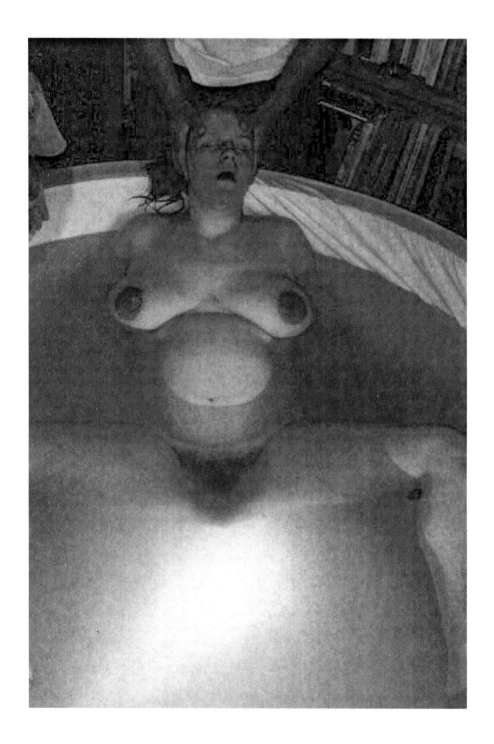

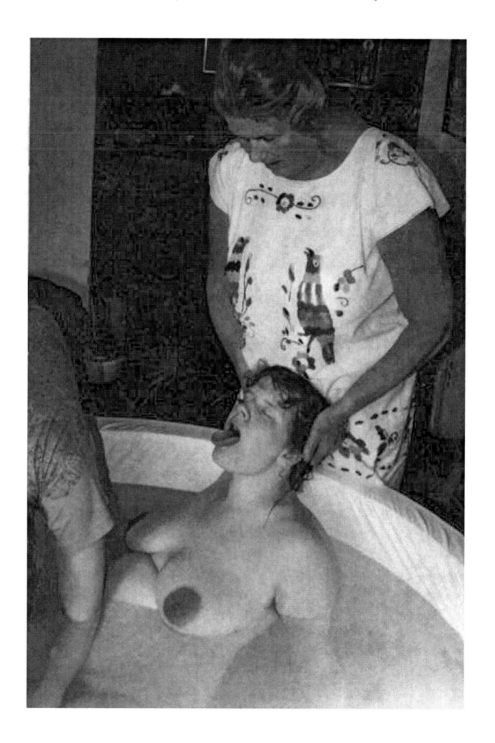

Supporting the woman while she's pushing

When the second stage of labour starts and the woman is pushing the baby out, she doesn't have to go to bed unless she wants to. She may have the ideal bed—a four-poster—and be able to squat holding on to one of the posts, or a bed with a solid headboard which she can grasp as she kneels facing it. If she is using a bed, it is best if the mattress is firm. But it may feel better to be on a clean sheet on the floor. Explore some of the positions she may want to use, as follows:

♥ She may want to stand with you behind her, holding her elbows, wrists or hands—whichever is most comfortable. If you are taller than her, keep a straight back, bending your knees slightly.

♥ She may want to stand in front of, facing you, with her hands clasped around your neck.

♥ She may prefer to sit upright between your legs (while you sit behind her) with her knees drawn up and legs well apart. (If you use this position, use pillows as necessary for extra support for you both.)

Being flexible

With all your preparations together, however, you will need to be flexible so that the labouring woman can do whatever feels right at the time of birth, even if it is not what she planned. It is important for you to know when to be silent, when to give the mother-to-be her own space, when not to intrude and to let her flow with the labour.

The power of birth is like the strength of water cascading in a mighty rush down a hillside. It is the power of seas and tides, the power of mountains moving. There is no way of ignoring it. A labouring woman cannot fight it. No amount of technique can enable her to be in control of it as she might be in control of a car or a computer. You should aim not to manage, conduct or coach her through this experience, but rather to give her strength and confidence as she allows her body to open and her baby to press through it to life.

Birth partner Q&A:

Q: Should a birth partner attend antenatal classes?

A: Yes. During classes your partner will learn ways of getting 'in tune' with your contractions and helping you to conserve your energy. In some classes, he or she will have a chance to rehearse supporting you and find out which forms of support are likely to suit you best. When you work with your birth partner in a group with other couples, you will learn a great deal about your birth partner and he or she will also learn much more about you. You'll also be able to share ideas with other people in the group.

Q: What sort of encouragement should I be given?

A: It often helps if he or she uses words that were used in the classes—those that held the most meaning for you both. They can be very simple, such as "Open", "Release", "Lovely", "Good" or repeated phrases, such as "Let it flow", "You're strong", "You're doing really well", "That's another one gone" or "We're getting there."

Q: I've heard that a partner should 'coach' a woman in labour. Is this what my birth partner ought to do?

A: No woman wants to be hectored or cajoled while she's in labour. If your birth partner offers you help without empathy, it can seem as if he or she is taking over and you may find yourself thinking: "Who's having this baby—you or me?!" For this reason, it's a good idea for your birth partner to use as few words as possible.

Q: What's the most important thing my birth partner can do?

A: Your birth partner can be your anchor in a stormy sea. Remaining calmly confident is the single most important quality he or she will need. Whatever techniques your birth partner learns—massage and offering strong physical support, so you can move around, for example—the essence of what he or she gives you will be warmth, which will come from being your lover or friend. He or she is certainly not a midwife, barefoot doctor, or coach.

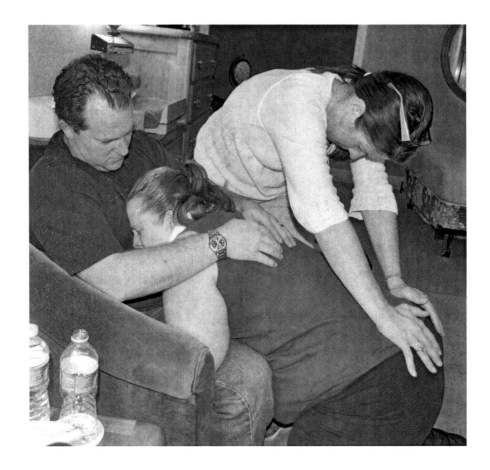

Sharing the experience

Having a strong support group, sharing the experience of pregnancy, swapping your accounts of interviews with obstetricians, hospital visits, and previous labours, and dealing with the medical system can help you discover what your rights are and learn effective strategies. You may want to be alone in labour. On the other hand, you may want to have close friends or family with you to increase your confidence and give comfort.

THE NEED FOR SUPPORT

When you plan a birth outside hospital, it helps to have a network of supporters—other couples and women—with whom you can share experiences, develop effective strategies for coping, and work together towards change.

> It helps to have a network of supporters with whom you can share experiences, develop effective strategies for coping, and work together towards change

You will probably find other like-minded people in your antenatal class, among your midwife's other clients and in childbirth organisations (see those listed in 'Useful contacts' on page 293). If you are having a baby in a birth centre you will be able to talk to newly delivered women and their partners over a cup of tea in the kitchen when you visit and will soon find that you are part of a group of prospective and new parents who support the birth centre. In the same way the groups formed to defend birth centres, midwifery-led units or GP units that are threatened with closure, in countries where the policy is one of centralisation, are strongly cohesive and militant in a very positive, celebratory way, and you will make new friends and discover many others who think as you do.

> A woman who wants a home birth tends to be isolated

In most countries a woman who wants a home birth tends to be isolated, she has to fight a lonely battle and may be treated by doctors as if she is suffering from severe emotional problems. Sometimes a hospital obstetrician has gone so far as to threaten a woman with psychiatric detention or with having her newborn baby confiscated because of her 'irresponsibility'. It is too much to expect a woman to be able to handle this hostility alone. In her book, *Midwives and Medical Men* (Heinemann, 1990), Jean Donnison says of women seeking home birth that they need "the patience of Job, the courage of Joan of Arc, and the political skill of a Metternich."[1]

66 We were sure that we didn't want to have our child come into a group of strangers, but rather into the loving circle of family and friends in a familiar setting.

SUPPORT FROM OTHER WOMEN

Traditionally, a woman in childbirth has always had other women helping her. As well as the midwife, there were friends, family members and neighbours who gave emotional and practical support. In 1658 Ralph Josselin recorded in his diary that his wife's labour had been so quick that, besides the midwife and nurse (for the baby), "only two or three women more got to her but God supplied all: young Mrs Harlakenden got up to us very speedily, and some others."[2]

Other women still give support to women in childbirth in most developing countries. When anthropologists are present at a birth, it is often quite difficult for them to find out who exactly the midwife is because she is one of a group of women helpers engaged in a task within a non-medical context. Childbirth is like bread-baking, laundering or cheese-making activities, that involve a community of women working together. In our own past, and cross-culturally, every adult woman was expected to know what to do in childbirth and how to help other women. She might have a recipe for a strengthening broth to be taken during labour, herbs to stimulate the uterus, or a lodestone (a naturally-occurring magnetic stone) or charm to help the birth go well.

66 *I'd never had that feeling so strongly before, of women sharing a process they understood and in complete harmony with each other. It was like a dance in which you all hear the same music and move accordingly, without having to talk about it.*

In medieval Europe, when a woman started labour she called on other women in the neighbourhood, who came bringing food to sustain them all during the labour and for celebration after the birth, and plenty of strong drink. Men were turned out of the house as women took over. These women would later testify at the baptism of the child and were known as 'God sibs', literally 'sisters in God'. Men must have resented this female takeover, and in English the word 'God sib' was gradually changed by men to 'gossip'.[3]

> In medieval Europe, when a woman started labour
> she called on other women in the neighbourhood

In pioneer times in North America, women relied heavily on what was known in Canada as 'turnabout' help

In pioneer times in North America, women relied heavily on what was known in Canada as 'turnabout' help. It carried on the old European tradition but with a new urgency, since many people were in isolated communities. Women had to be able to heal illness, mend bones, comfort the dying and help one another in childbirth. When a baby was on the way, they made each other baby clothes and sewed beautiful bed quilts. Then, when labour started, they cooked meals, did the housework, took over the woman's other duties, such as milking the cows, and cared for the mother and her family for some days after the birth, until she was fit to take up again the heavy work that was an integral part of life on a pioneer farm.[4]

These women often travelled some distance between their own homes, where they had work of their own to do, and the new mother's home. And, if a woman went into labour when the helper was in the middle of a major domestic project, the helper brought her own work along.

66 I recall one time a man coming 18 miles in a sleigh to take my grandmother to his wife who was expecting a baby. My grandmother had mixed bread dough earlier in the day, so she packed the pan of dough in with her in this sleigh, which was comfortably warm with lots of blankets and quilts and heated stones. When she arrived at the farmer's home, the dough had risen enough to bake, so she baked it in the stove in his kitchen and, after she delivered the baby, the husband drove my grandmother back home with all her bread baked.[5]

There was rarely any exchange of money for this kind of 'turnabout' help. Families repaid each other with gifts of produce, assistance with farm work, or with building and equipping a house. The strong links forged between women at times of great significance in their lives formed a basis for the new communities that were being created.

There was rarely any exchange of money for 'turnabout' help. Families repaid each other with gifts or help of another kind.

Postnatal support was given as a matter of course too, and women sent over cooked meals for the new mother and her family. As one midwife in an isolated fishing community in Newfoundland put it: "There was always other women from around coming and looking out to things that needed to be done. No one starved, let me tell you, when a woman was lyin' in."[6] In this community it was the custom on the last day of lying in to have an 'up-sitting day', when the neighbouring women, together with the midwife, gathered in the new mother's house for tea and 'Groaning Cake', often baked by the father.[7]

In the past no woman had to labour alone or among strangers

In the past no woman had to labour alone or among strangers, and no mother lacked postnatal nurture. Isolation and loneliness came with the move from home to hospital. Even in hospital, having another woman there who is responsible to you, not to the hospital, and who has no medical function, may bring a great deal of comfort, ease labour and result in a better outcome. When research was done in Guatemala comparing the labours of women going into hospital with no support from other women with those of others who had one-to-one support from a caring woman, even one they did not know before, the results were spectacularly in favour of the woman-to-woman support.[8] A Canadian study found that those women who had their partners with them and had also been assigned a *monitrice* were admitted to hospital later in labour, were more likely to require no medication during childbirth, and to have an intact perineum.[9]

Booking a personal birth companion, a doula, is a way of rediscovering this woman-to-woman help. (See the Useful contacts on page 293.) You get to know each other during pregnancy and you call her when you start labour. She supports you and your partner if you have one and assists, but does not replace the midwife, and gives practical help and emotional support as long as you need it after the birth.

66 It mattered to me that the women there had had babies themselves and knew what it was like. They weren't shocked or surprised by anything. They stayed calm, down-to-earth and always comforting.

With home birth the presence of other women in the family and female friends occurs quite spontaneously without the need to obtain permission or worry about protocol. In such a setting women rediscover an ancient role during childbirth and the postpartum weeks. They can form a strong, loving group to nurture the mother and be in company with her through a significant life transition.

Doctors often find the presence of other women during a birth very threatening to their professional status. Hospital nurses and midwives may feel uneasy in the same way. They fear that they will lose control of the patient. So in a hospital you may be told that there is 'no room', or that other women might 'get in the way' or distract you and make the labour go badly.

GETTING THE RIGHT KIND OF HELP

It is undoubtedly true that a lively party going on around you during labour may prove irritating, and contradictory advice or general chat can be as intrusive, in its own way, as obstetric intervention. Any women who are with you should be able to tune in to how you are feeling and what you want of them. Michel Odent believes that the presence of other people, even the husband, may prevent a woman from trusting her instincts and from 'being on another planet', as he calls the state of focused inward concentration when labour is at its height.

But when women are bonded together in a task—whether in a workplace outside the home, a kitchen, or a birth room—there is a special quality about the work they do. There is a common give-and-take in their interaction, an understanding that develops between them—often with no need for words—that can be described only by the word 'sisterhood'. I am not claiming that something similar cannot exist for men too—only that childbirth is a female task and that women sharing in the spirit of birthing create an atmosphere that can give huge strength and confidence to the labouring woman.

There should be no talking during contractions, no bustling about or busyness, only a turning towards the woman in labour. She should be at the centre of everything that is happening and her needs and wishes are paramount. If she wants to be alone, her helpers leave and wait nearby. If she wants only one other person with her after all, that is her choice. There must be no conflict, no domineering attitudes, no competition to give her most help. Those present are simply watching and waiting on life.

ENSURING SUPPORT FOR THE MIDWIFE

It is also vital that there is at least one person in the group who is quietly supporting the midwife. This is especially the case in any country where home birth is perceived by most doctors as a dangerous gamble. The midwife may need somewhere to lie down and rest if labour is slow, may welcome food and drink and perhaps a bath. She also needs strong emotional support and to know that her work is appreciated, and that she is valued as a person.

> During labour and birth it is vital that there is no friction between those present and that there is at least one person in the group who is quietly supporting the midwife

An English midwife, Caroline Flint, has written: "To work as a midwife is stressful because, to work effectively and sensitively, the midwife gives so much of herself, and she becomes so involved with and such a part of the family with which she is involved. To enable her to be a fount of such strength, a source of so much comfort, she herself must have support and cherishing!"[10]

66 I felt close to her. There was that wonderful 'with woman' feeling.

When one of my daughters was giving birth in our home, using a birthing pool, the second stage was very gentle and was taking a long time. I was aware that both midwives were rather tired. I went to make a pot of tea to refresh us. The senior midwife came in and said, "Sheila, you are really confident that Tess can do this, aren't you?" We looked each other in the eyes. "Yes, I am. I have complete confidence in her." She smiled. "That's all right then," she replied, and went back to help the unfolding of this new life with increased confidence. It culminated in the triumphant birth in water of a 4.75kg (10½lb) vigorous baby, whose mother had an intact perineum and next to no bleeding. As Tess lifted her new son up in her arms, he looked up at her, turned to us and then back to her, and smiled.

> To work as a midwife is stressful... she gives so much of herself

During those hours of labour there were two midwives, both dear friends of mine, Tess's husband Jon and myself, with my husband, unobtrusively taking photographs. Tess clung to Jon physically, but with each late-first-stage contraction she sought the eyes of one midwife, while the other cradled her head in a way that made her feel utterly safe. At times one of us passed her a small sponge on which to suck, brushed her hair back from her face, or gave her iced water to sip. Sometimes I held her head and the midwife and Jon held her legs. Then Jon and I held her legs and the midwife her head. And when she was out of the water she often squatted or knelt, with the midwife and her husband on either side with their arms around her and the other midwife face to face with her, giving her understanding and love.

Afterwards the senior midwife told me that when she worked on the delivery suite in the hospital in the days following she felt very alone, even though midwives there are supposed to work as members of teams. Even in a large institution where people are milling about—and perhaps *especially* in a large institution—a midwife can feel unsupported. The support that other women can give a midwife in an out-of-hospital birth is precious.

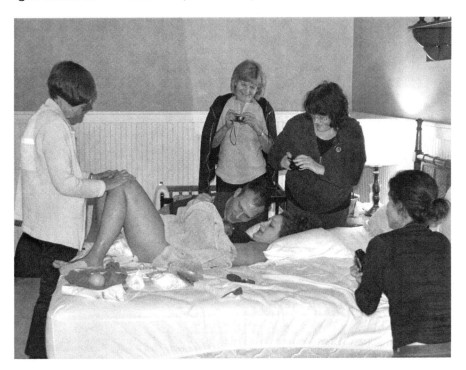

CHILDREN

Many women who already have children choose an out-of-hospital birth so that the older siblings can share in the birth experience, meet the new baby in an atmosphere that is warmer and more welcoming than that of a hospital, and not have to be separated from their mother. Yet there is more to it even than that. All of us who approach childbirth with no idea of what happens, except what can be gained from books and films, are deprived. Girls growing up without any awareness of what it feels like to give birth, other than the fear of pain and injury, are especially deprived. In medicalising childbirth and removing it from the home, our culture has made birth, like dying, a fearful ordeal that can be dealt with only by experts; it is no longer part of our shared lives and is out of women's control. In bringing birth back into a setting that is controlled by women, making it a family occasion and involving the children, we reclaim it and prepare children to reclaim it for themselves.

66 Holding in her arms a newborn who is still crumpled, warm and wet from the womb helps an older child really feel that this is 'our' baby.

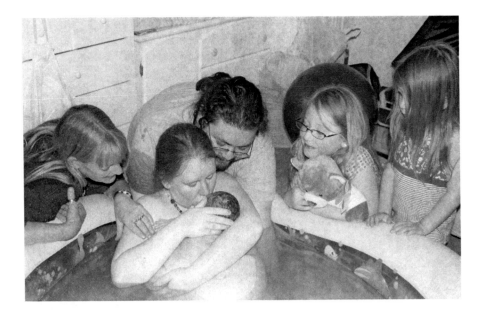

❝ There she was, wriggling and screaming! Chris lifted her into my arms. I realised my other three kids had missed her birth. Then there they were, in the room. Each of their faces, at that moment, is fixed in my mind for ever.

Don't sit a two-year-old down in front of you in labour and expect him to watch quietly even for 10 minutes, if what he really wants is to stampede around the garden in a boisterous game. He should be free to go in and out as he wishes, cuddle up beside you when he wants the comfort of your presence or is sleepy. He can help by offering you ice chips if your mouth is dry, or a damp cloth for your forehead to cool you down.

Women are often adamant that they would not want their older children present because it would be distracting and they would get in the way. They think they would have to be mothering when they want to concentrate on themselves. This is one effect of the isolation of women from each other. There is often no one else, apart from the mother, who understands what a small child wants or who can provide comfort. Nevertheless, having a child around when you are in labour works only if one of your helpers, someone close to you and whom your child loves, has special responsibility for him or her. Otherwise your birth partner will be constantly distracted from attending to your needs with changing a nappy, fetching a potty, finding the teddy bear, or kissing a hurt better. So plan ahead for this well before the time of birth and let your child share in your plans. If he or she is around when you are pushing the baby out, able to see what is happening, share in the excitement of birth, and let him or her touch and hold the new baby immediately afterwards. It will be an unforgettable experience.

❝ I agreed to look after Stephen (aged three) and take him out if he became bored. We went off and made gingerbread men in the kitchen, and then David called us back in because the baby was about to be born. She was pushing and we could soon see the crown of the baby's head. I explained what we were seeing and what was happening. With the next push the baby's head emerged. Stephen was enthralled! Soon after the baby was born, he sat in the armchair and cuddled her.

How can I prepare my child for the birth of this baby?

To prepare your child for the birth you may want to:

♥ Tell your child how he or she grew inside your body, looking together at photographs of fetal development.[11]

♥ Make a picture book together about when your older child was a baby, and tell the story of that birth in simple language.

♥ Look at photographs of new babies and talk about how they look, how they behave, and what they can do.

♥ Pack a bag with new colouring books, crayons, snacks and juice for each child.

♥ Watch an animal birth, or see a film of animals being born.

♥ Describe what happens during birth, and how the baby's head looks when it first appears. Help your child understand the appearance and function of the umbilical cord and the placenta, and distinguish clearly between birth blood and the blood of injury.

♥ Look together at birth photographs and talk about them.

♥ Have your child meet and, if possible, hold a new baby, and watch the mother breastfeeding. Talk about how a new baby needs to be cared for and why.

❝ Olivia is seven and begged not to be left out of it. She was sitting beside me when the baby's head was born, and leant over and kissed it and said, "Hello, baby!" I felt a wave of warmth and love for her and for everybody, and at the next push the baby slithered out. She was so excited! We all kissed and cuddled and cried with joy.

❝ My three-year-old son saw his brother being born. When he saw the baby coming, he sang, 'Happy birthday to you'.

Look at photos of new babies and talk about how they look

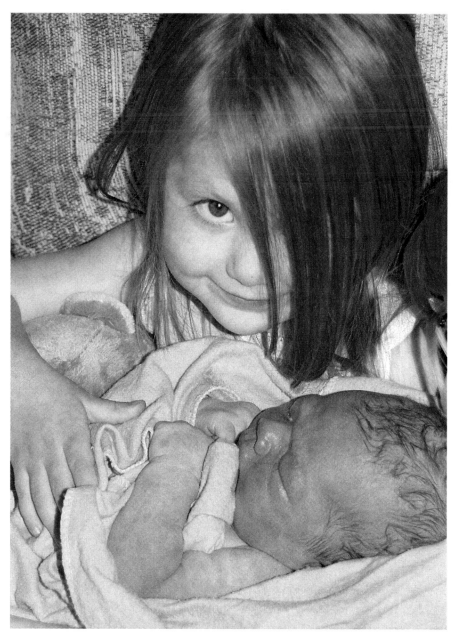

Remember that it is easy to overload a small child with information about birth and babies. This child wants to be the centre of your attention and not feel rejected in favour of the new baby. So you will also want to talk about feelings: feeling alone, feeling loved, feeling excited and feeling sad.

It is essential that your midwife knows your child too, so that she feels comfortable with the child's presence, and that the child knows her as a friend whose arrival is welcomed. They can develop a relationship during antenatal visits, when your midwife explains what she is doing and why, in simple language, and gets your child to 'help'. He or she will listen to the baby's heartbeats, which sound like galloping hooves, feel the baby kick, see you practise the different positions and movements you may want to use in labour, and watch you relaxing and breathing. It is a good idea to rehearse the noises you may want to make too, so that your child is not surprised by them: grunting, moaning, panting, sighing and groaning. Children usually take all this in their stride if they are well prepared and if they feel secure.

A child at a home birth is witness to the care and love that is given to the mother. This is an important learning experience about human compassion, sensitivity and tenderness. The child is witness also to the power in women, the energy in the mother, and the strength of women to help and support each other. And, if it turns out that way, the child is present as the miracle of life unfolds, hears the first cry, and sees warm, damp, crumpled flesh become a little person who can be held and stroked.

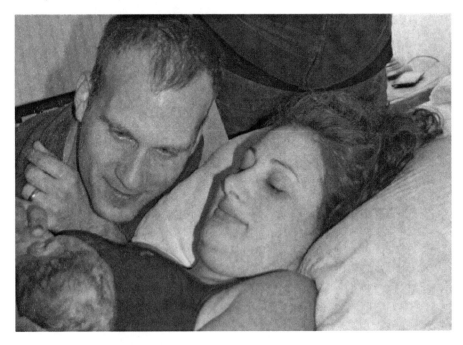

Other children Q&A:

Q: What do I tell my child about birth?

A: Be completely open and honest about the birth and make it exciting. "The baby grows inside a muscle bag in my body called 'the uterus'. When it is ready to be born my uterus squeezes tightly and gives the baby very big hugs. The opening of the bag gets bigger and bigger until the top of the baby's head can pass through, like when your head pushes through the neck of your sweater."

Q: How else can I prepare my child?

A: It is a good idea to rehearse the noises you may make, so that the child is not surprised by them: grunting, moaning, panting, sighing and groaning. This can be great fun! Plan ahead and let the child share your plans. An older child can make his or her own birth plan too: what to play with during labour, how to help you in simple ways, and what the party will be like after the baby is born.

Q: Should I ask someone to be there to look after my child?

A: Having a child around when you are in labour works only if someone has special responsibility for the child. Otherwise, your birth partner will be constantly distracted from attending to your needs with changing a nappy, fetching a potty, finding the teddy bear, or kissing a hurt better.

Q: Should my child watch the birth?

A: You know your child best. It depends a lot on your feelings at the time, too. Don't sit a two-year-old in front of you in labour and expect him or her to watch quietly if what he or she really wants is to stampede around the garden. Your child should be free to go in and out and cuddle up beside you when he or she wants the comfort of your presence, or is sleepy.

Q: Could the experience be overwhelming?

A: Children usually take birth in their stride if they are well prepared and feel secure.

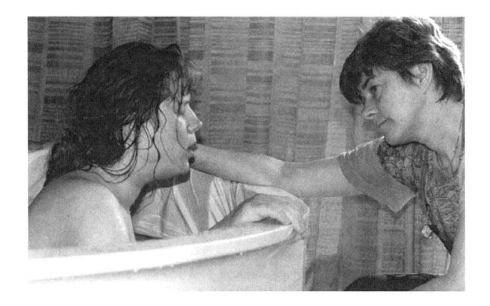

Meeting challenges

All that is needed for most labours to go well is a healthy, pregnant woman who has loving support in labour, self-confidence, and attendants with infinite patience. Sadly, most of us don't have these things, and then even a straightforward labour can become difficult, with rescue manoeuvres taking the place of the nurturing that is the basis of good midwifery care. Women who have their babies in hospital are more likely to have difficult labours because they are in hospital. The physiology of birth has been disturbed. They are also at risk of suffering the effects of iatrogenic medical care—that is, being subjected to interventions that themselves introduce pathology. This is not to say that problems never develop in planned out-of-hospital births, only that they can usually be solved by simple, non-invasive measures.

QUESTIONS YOU MIGHT BE WONDERING ABOUT

In this chapter I look at what can be done when difficulties are encountered, so that you and your midwife can discuss together what action to take.

What if I'm overdue?

> ❝ Kathryn was originally due on 12 September, but she was born on 20 October. I was allowed to go for so long overdue as it was decided that I had not conceived until four weeks after my last period. I had only one period after coming off the Pill, and the cycle had not returned to normal.

Most babies are not born on the date they are expected. Generally speaking, it is safer for them to be born after the expected date than preterm. Although with prolonged pregnancy every hour may seem like a week, and each week a month, a baby will usually be born within 10 days of the expected date. If you go past 10 days, it may be because you had a long menstrual cycle, ovulated later than you thought, and so conceived later, or because the date based on an ultrasound scan that you were given was incorrect. Gestational age based on the known first day of the last menstruation is sometimes more accurate than ultrasound.[1]

There is an unexplained stillbirth rate of 1 in 1,000 babies at 40 weeks. This starts to go up at 41 weeks, when it is 1.2 per 1,000 births. At 42 weeks it is 1.3 per 1,000 births. So there seems to be no advantage in inducing labour before 40 weeks unless the baby is obviously not doing well in the uterus.[2]

Going for bumpy car rides or drinking gin does not start labour. Uncomfortable journeys just leave you tired and aching. Alcohol inhibits labour. Alcohol used to be given to stop preterm labour because it prevents secretion by the pituitary gland of oxytocin, the natural substance that initiates labour. Alcohol may cause respiratory depression in the newborn.[3]

Going for bumpy car rides or drinking gin does not start labour—
uncomfortable journeys just leave you tired and aching

Can I help myself go into labour?

You may find that contractions start after sexual stimulation, which leads to the release of oxytocin in the bloodstream. This may have an effect similar to that of synthetic oxytocin administered through an intravenous drip in order to start labour artificially. Even what is for many women the very gentle arousal produced by nipple stimulation (carried out by you or someone else) may produce contractions, if continued for 20 minutes or so at a time.[4] Stroke the nipples with your fingers, rolling, sucking or licking them, or rest a warm face cloth on your breasts, lifting it off when it cools, dipping it in hot water, and pressing it against the nipples again.

> You may find that contractions start after sexual stimulation, which leads to the release of oxytocin in the bloodstream

Contractions may at first be very short and only gradually become longer, although in some women long, strong contractions are stimulated immediately. If they last for one minute or longer, reduce or stop the stimulation, since you may be particularly sensitive to it.

As you stimulate one nipple, you will notice that both nipples react, and may be aware of sensations in the other breast too. The same happens when you breastfeed. When the baby sucks at one breast, the milk ejection reflex occurs in both.

> There is an extraordinary link between the nipples and the uterus, as you discover when you breastfeed.

There is an extraordinary link between the nipples and the uterus, as you discover when you breastfeed. In the days after birth, when the baby latches on, you experience the warm, buzzing, milk ejection reflex as blood rushes into your breasts and, either at the same time or soon after as the baby sucks, you experience strong contractions of the uterus. These can be quite painful in the early days but they are useful because they speed up your uterus's return to its pre-pregnancy size and shape.

> When the baby latches on, you experience the warm, buzzing, milk ejection reflex... and strong contractions of the uterus

Sexual intercourse may also stimulate contractions. This is because of the combined effect of oxytocin release and semen in the vagina. Semen is rich in prostaglandins. In fact, it is the richest source in the human body. Synthetic prostaglandins are used for induction in the form of a gel or pessary inserted in the cervix. To be most effective, semen should form a pool around the cervix— so back to the missionary position! Lie still for half an hour after your partner has ejaculated, so that the semen collects round the cervix. During this time your partner can caress your breasts so that you have both forms of stimulation.

Some years ago the Japanese invented a whirring machine that could be inserted against the cervix to start contractions, because it was found that local stimulation of the tissues was effective for induction. In the absence of such a machine, and perhaps in preference to it (because of the possibility of infection), you might explore the effect of lying on your back with your ankles on your partner's shoulders so that his penis can be introduced deeply. This is not comfortable and should be done very, very gently. A clean finger could be used to tickle the cervix gently instead.

You can experience sexual arousal without a partner, of course. Masturbation will produce contractions and, because it is possible to have an orgasm very quickly, and to experience multiple orgasm, with self-stimulation, it may be more effective than intercourse in starting off labour.

Although breast or clitoral stimulation does not always get labour going, it may well ripen your cervix, making it soft, flexible and thinned out, so that it dilates more easily when labour really does start.

❝ My doctor was muttering about induction. So we went to bed early and decided to try your method of natural induction. Contractions started, like cramps, about 10 minutes after we made love and Neil kept them going by playing with my nipples while I dozed off... I came to about 3 o'clock in the morning when contractions were coming about every five minutes. Neil was half-asleep but had one hand on the top of my tummy to feel contractions, and kept twiddling my nipple with the other. He felt very pleased with himself.

What if I stop feeling my baby moving around inside me?

If you go past your due date, it may be reassuring to make a note of fetal movements. A baby who is moving vigorously is fine.

Although a baby makes fewer whole-body movements in the last few weeks of pregnancy, because it is a tight fit in the uterus, a healthy baby continues to kick, often when you are resting or lying in the bath. You can select a time of day when your baby is always at its most active and monitor what is happening during that time.

If you find that your baby has quietened down, the most likely possibility is that labour is about to start in this case. There may be other signs:

♥ a rush of energy as you feel the 'nesting' instinct and want to clean out cupboards or finish a work project

♥ the need to empty your bladder frequently

♥ slight looseness of the bowels—like a minor digestive upset

♥ low backache

♥ a feeling that your baby's head is hanging between your legs like a coconut

♥ more frequent Braxton Hicks (practice) contractions of your uterus

When fetal movements are much reduced and labour does not start, there is a chance that a baby is no longer being nourished well by the placenta. You will want to check on this, so ring your midwife, say what has happened and ask for fetal heart monitoring.

You can enjoy these last unanticipated days of pregnancy with special activities for which otherwise you will never have time—that restaurant you meant to try, the concert you thought you wouldn't be able to go to because the baby would just be born, a day with a friend, a picnic, a trip to an art gallery or museum, or a play or film that you can fit in now. Don't just sit and wait for the first twinges and brood over what seems by now to be an elephant pregnancy. Soon there will be a baby in your arms.

You can enjoy these last unanticipated days of pregnancy with special activities which otherwise you will never have time for

What can I do if I think labour has started, but it hasn't?

Many women have painful contractions that might be the start of labour in the last few weeks, before they actually go into labour. This is 'prodromal' labour, and means that changes are taking place in preparation for labour before dilation starts. It is a sign that contractions are beginning to soften and thin out the cervix and push down the baby's presenting part—the part of the baby nearest your cervix, usually the head. Although tiring, this may reduce the length of time you are in labour.

You may be told that you are in 'false' labour. This does not mean that you are telling lies or that your body is not working properly. What you are feeling is real. Contractions occur especially at night and may keep you awake; they may be quite regular for several hours. The problem with prodromal labour is that a woman is likely to be in a permanently alert state, waiting for further action. This is very tiring and results in a lowering of morale even before she feels regular contractions that dilate the cervix.

If this happens to you, it is important to get some sleep, perhaps with a special bedtime ritual: soaking in a bath with lavender oil and then having a hot drink or a small glass of wine, and listening to soothing music as you settle down.

What if my waters break before labour starts?

10% of women have premature rupture of the membranes at term (when the baby is due), and 8 out of 10 of these start labour spontaneously within 12 hours,[5] although sometimes a woman has to wait as long as 24 hours before it begins. Premature rupture is more likely when there have been vaginal examinations in the weeks preceding,[6] so this is a good reason for declining such examinations in the last weeks of pregnancy.

When your waters break there may be a gush of fluid or a slow trickle. If there is only a dribble it is probably the hindwaters (the part of the bubble behind the baby's head) that are leaking, and they often reseal themselves after a while. You can ignore this. If there is a gush of fluid, note whether the fluid is clear, or stained brown or green. If it is clear and your baby is already engaged in your pelvis, you do not need to take special action. If it is stained, the baby has emptied its bowels of meconium, a sign that it could be under stress. You should call your midwife so that the baby's position can be checked.

Often any meconium present is not fresh, which is a sign that the baby was stressed some time ago. If your baby is breech, meconium is squeezed out mechanically as the bottom is pressed down and this is not an indication that the baby is stressed.

Premature rupture of the membranes is sometimes taken as a sign that a woman is going to have a more difficult labour. But this is not so. There is no such thing as a 'dry' labour, because fresh amniotic fluid is created that keeps the baby, its cord and the surrounding tissues moist.

An important thing to know when membranes rupture is the position in which your baby is lying, so it is helpful to be aware of this at the end of pregnancy. If the baby is head down and the head is low in the pelvis, there is no possibility of the type of emergency occurring when a loop of cord slips down beneath the head. There is a remote chance of this happening if the head is still high, however, or if the baby is lying in a less usual position—breech or transverse (across the uterus). Once your membranes have ruptured, do not put anything inside your vagina or you may introduce infection. There should be no vaginal examinations out of curiosity either. The more vaginal examinations that take place, the greater the risk of infection.

If you wait anxiously for the first contraction, you will be tired out by the time your energy is really needed. So put on a sanitary pad—change it regularly—and go to bed and sleep, do some gentle work around the house or garden, play cards or a good board game, listen to music, or watch television.

To check there is no infection, take your temperature every three to four hours. If there is infection you become slightly feverish and you should let your caregiver know this. When you empty your bowels, be careful to wipe from front to back, away from your vagina, so that you do not introduce bacteria from your rectum. Don't starve yourself during this wait. You may not want to eat once labour starts, so avoid a long fast now. Have plenty of fluids—fruit juice, tea, or whatever you fancy—to help replace your amniotic fluid, and keep your energy up with snacks of high-carbohydrate food, such as pasta, baked potato, and pancakes with syrup. Some midwives suggest taking supplementary Vitamin C to build resistance to infection—250mg every few hours.[7]

To check there is no infection, take your temperature every three to four hours. If you get slightly feverish, let your caregiver know

What if the cord prolapses?

A prolapsed cord is an obstetric emergency. It occurs rarely—in 0.3% of pregnancies. It happens occasionally in late pregnancy, when membranes rupture prematurely, whether or not a woman intends to have her baby in hospital. Prolapse is dangerous because the baby's oxygen supply depends on blood flowing freely through the cord. When it prolapses, the cord gets nipped between the mother's pelvis and the baby's presenting part (head or bottom). A caesarean section is often the only way to deliver the baby safely.

> A prolapsed cord is an obstetric emergency—
> but it occurs in only 0.3% of pregnancies

Your midwife will diagnose that the baby's cord is trapped if it can be felt pulsating in your vagina, but sometimes it is too high to feel and the clue is a marked deceleration in the fetal heartbeat immediately following membrane rupture when the presenting part was high. Go to hospital immediately.

Emergency treatment is to get into a knee-chest position with your bottom high in the air. Your midwife, or your birth partner if no professional caregiver is present, inserts two clean fingers into your cervix to press the baby's presenting part up and away from the cord. If you go to hospital in a car or ambulance, keep in this position with a blanket thrown over you, your pelvis raised high on a beanbag or pile of pillows, and your helper's fingers maintaining pressure inside your cervix to lift the presenting part away from it. An alternative is for your midwife to introduce 400ml to 700ml of saline into your bladder to cushion the cord. This slows down uterine activity for a while too.

> A prolapsed cord is very unlikely to occur during a home birth or
> in any birth place where invasive procedures are not practised

A prolapsed cord is very unlikely to occur during a home birth or in any birth place where invasive procedures are not practised. It is usually a consequence of intervention—rupturing the membranes artificially when the presenting part is high.

> A prolapsed cord is usually a consequence of intervention—
> rupturing the membranes when the presenting part is high

How can I handle a long, slow labour?

It is difficult to time the onset of labour precisely and, although some women are suddenly aware that this is IT, far more women experience a gentle lead-in to labour. You may decide you are in labour with contractions that are spaced about 10 minutes from the start of one to the start of the next, or may adopt a 'wait-and-see' attitude. Anxiety makes a woman more sensitive to the pre-labour phase and alerts her to action before she can do anything to help herself. It is better to relax and let things happen. Your body will tell you that you are in labour when it really needs your concentrated attention.

The shortest labours are not necessarily the best. A rapid labour can be shocking for the mother and prove stressful for the baby. In statistical terms the best outcomes follow a labour of between 12 and 24 hours for women having their first babies, and a labour lasting between 3 and 24 hours for women having subsequent babies.[8]

Slow dilation is completely normal for some women. The arbitrary decision made by obstetricians who practise 'active management' that labour must not last longer than 12 hours, or that dilation must proceed by 1cm per hour, puts the woman under stress and makes her attendants anxious too, so that they sometimes act unwisely in an attempt to hurry labour along. They may rupture the membranes in order to hasten a slow labour. But if this is done before 4cm dilation of the cervix it can actually slow down an already slow labour. If you are already around 9cm dilated, however—the point at which membranes usually rupture naturally—amniotomy may speed up the late first stage.[9]

In hospital a long, slow labour is often termed 'failure to progress' only because caregivers find the waiting intolerable. There is an art in adapting to a long labour and not being hassled or discouraged.

66 Ross and I decided to take the dog for a vigorous walk in the park to see if we could hurry things along. It was a real pleasure, interrupted by strong contractions that began coming every 10 minutes again. I sat down, or leaned against him or a tree, and he supported me through the breathing. I felt strong and confident.

Woman having a hospital birth:

" If someone doesn't cover that clock, I'm going to break it!

Here are some more tips for helping you handle a long labour...

♥ Intersperse activity and rest, and change your activities frequently. Avoid boredom. Bake a cake for the celebration afterwards, soak in a bath, go for a walk, sew or knit—anything rather than lying in bed wondering if there is something wrong because labour is not going faster.

♥ Eat easily digested, smooth foods, such as potato puree, soup, mashed banana, ice cream, sorbet, honey sandwiches or yogurt, and drink plenty of fluids. In most cultures special foods are used to keep up a woman's strength in labour. In Pakistan it may be a paste of dates and sesame seeds; in China chicken ginger soup; in Colombia fig juice; and in the Caribbean spice tea which, like the raspberry leaf tea popular in Europe, has a mild oxytocic action.

♥ Move around and keep changing position to stimulate uterine activity, and to encourage the baby to descend and rotate with the crown of the head against your cervix. Rock your pelvis, go up and down stairs, and lunge against the wall.

♥ Soak in a bath or have a shower to refresh you and help you relax.

♥ Empty your bladder every hour and a half to two hours. (Your partner can keep a note of it and remind you.)

♥ A woman in slow labour welcomes quiet, calm reassurance: "You are doing well. The baby is fine. It doesn't matter that labour is slow." You should not feel under any pressure of time. It is often good to be left alone with your birth partner.

♥ Explore what happens when you do nipple stimulation or gentle clitoral massage. You can do it yourself or ask your partner to do it. Or you could both get into bed, send everyone away, turn off the light, and have a cuddle for an hour.

A midwife talking about a client's labour:

66 We spent much of the first stage in the garden, putting in bedding plants together. Then we came in and made some biscuits and cleared up the kitchen. By that time I could tell from her breathing that she was nearly fully dilated.

What if I have a start-stop labour?

66 Contractions stopped completely. I was so disappointed. I felt ready to cry. So I did cry, long and hard. John and I barbecued the biggest steak we could find and ate lots of salad and vegetables and potatoes to keep it company. I put an apple sauce cake in the oven and got ready for bed. Then I felt a strong contraction and, after that, another one...

I lay down for a couple of hours, and my contractions spaced out more. Then I got up again and found that, with walking, the intensity increased and they came every three or four minutes, lasting 45 to 60 seconds.

Some labours are slow in a different way. They start and then seem to stop. The uterus contracts weakly or ceases to contract for an interval, then starts again, but may have another phase of inactivity. There may be plateaux like this when nothing much seems to be happening.

A woman in slow labour welcomes quiet, calm reassurance. Be aware that the uterus is very responsive to anxiety.

A start-stop labour occurs most commonly when a woman is admitted to hospital and her previous regular, strong contractions become spasmodic and weak. The cause is anxiety. The uterus is very responsive to anxiety and this is as true for other mammals as for women. Interference can make any animal's labour more difficult. For example, when mice are disturbed during labour, their labours are prolonged and they are more likely to deliver dead pups.[10]

If you have a start-stop labour, try to find out why you're anxious. Bring it out into the open and ask others to help you deal with it.

If you have a start-stop labour, try to find why you are anxious. Bring it out into the open and ask your birth partner and midwife to help you deal with it. Before you can melt into your labour, you are going to have to discard all these fears.

Keep active, unless you are very tired, in which case rest in a darkened room, perhaps with soft music to screen you from any disturbing sounds. Your midwife can rest near you, and many midwives bring some sewing or other work to do ready for just such eventualities.

Keep active, unless you are very tired, in which case
rest in a darkened room, perhaps with soft music
to screen you from any disturbing sounds

There is a physical cause for some start-stop labours—for example, the baby's head is in an awkward position and becomes stuck. Your midwife will monitor the fetal heart regularly and assess the situation. When a baby is awkwardly positioned, moving about and rocking and rolling your pelvis may coax it into a better position so that labour can progress. And even when the head is a tight fit and the baby's descent through the pelvis is delayed, the spontaneous movements a woman makes can assist the uterus to ease the baby's head through the cervix and down the birth canal.

The diagnosis of cephalo-pelvic disproportion (CPD) is made far too often, when what is really meant is, "We couldn't be bothered to wait," or "We were afraid," or "The mother's morale dropped." If, after discussion and exploring alternative ways of stimulating labour, you decide that further action is called for, you will need to go to hospital. An oxytocin intravenous drip (syntocinon) cannot be set up at home because it is a powerful and potentially dangerous intervention. For some labours it is the most effective solution to reduced uterine activity. A stop-start or slow labour is not an emergency, however, and you will have time to discuss it fully and come to a decision with your midwife.

The diagnosis of CPD is made far too often, when
what is really meant is, "We couldn't be bothered to wait,"
or "We were afraid," or "The mother's morale dropped."

How can I deal with backache?

One of the most difficult things to handle in labour is low backache. It continues as a gnawing ache between contractions, as well as being a sharp sacro-lumbar pain during them, and can wear down any woman's spirits. Backache occurs particularly when the baby's back is against the mother's spine (posterior position) and the hard back of the baby's extended head (that is, when the chin is lifted) is pressing against her sacrum and sacro-lumbar ligaments. Any position in which the baby is tipped forwards on to the mother's abdominal wall and away from her spine may ease it: a forward-kneeling or all-fours position, for example, together with swinging, rocking, and circling of the pelvis. Tipping the baby forwards also helps it to rotate from the posterior to the anterior position. The baby is more likely to tuck its head in and turn against the abdominal muscles, especially if they are relaxed, than against the bony spine.

Firm massage or counterpressure over the painful area is also helpful. Hot or cold compresses relieve pain, too. Either a hot water bottle or a small packet of frozen peas may work well. A strong jet of hot or cold water directed on to the spot as pain builds up often brings relief. Some women labouring in water find that massage while they are in a forward-leaning position in the pool provides amazing pain relief.

> Any position in which the baby is tipped forwards on to the mother's abdominal wall, away from her spine, may ease pain

Transcutaneous electronic nerve stimulation (TENS) helps some women, but proves irritating or ineffective for others. TENS is done with a handheld instrument, about the size of a camera, which sends electrical impulses to the brain to block pain messages. It is battery operated, with four electrodes which are attached with adhesive tape at either side of the spine, two with their upper edges at the level of the lower ribs and two in the lower back. You control its operation yourself and can move about, lie down, or sit up. It seems to be less effective for abdominal than for back pain.

> Firm massage or counterpressure over the painful area is also helpful. Hot or cold compresses relieve pain too.

The instrument's low frequency current produces a buzzing sensation, which stimulates the release of natural (endogenous) opiates and endorphins into the cerebro-spinal fluid, thus raising tolerance of pain and increasing the sense of wellbeing.[11] If you know before the onset of labour that your baby is posterior, it can be worth getting hold of TENS equipment. It is something you can do to help yourself, and is harmless to the baby.[12]

Any woman with severe backache needs her helpers' undivided attention and encouragement to keep going. Because pain of this kind is very wearing, she may feel unable to move about. If this happens to you, flop forwards, spreadeagled over a beanbag, so that your partner can reach your back and massage or press against it. The position will help the baby's head to rotate. Or lie on your side with the arm which is underneath spread out behind you, your limbs well flexed, and your head bent forwards. You will spontaneously select the correct side on which to lie, because it is more comfortable. Most posterior babies lie with their back on the mother's right side: the right occipito posterior (ROP) position. This is five times more common than left occipito posterior (LOP). If your baby is ROP, lie on your left side with your top knee drawn up and pressing against your abdomen. This encourages the baby to tip forwards into a position where it is easier for it to turn to the anterior. If your baby is LOP, you will be more comfortable on your right side, and this helps the baby turn. In this position, your birth partner can sit close against your lower back, with the side of his pelvis pressing hard against the area where you feel most pain. You will find the right spot after a little experimentation. Then you can have the whole weight of his body leaning against you at the peak of pain. He can also massage your back by rocking his own pelvis.

You will find the right spot with a little experimentation

Once the baby rotates, backache may vanish almost miraculously and you go straight into the pushing stage. When I was doing anthropological field work in Jamaica, I found that the shape of many women's pelvises was such that their babies were posterior for a long time in labour. They disliked the backache but welcomed it as a sign that the 'gate' in their backs was creaking open to let the baby out. If you think of that pain as a gate opening, it may be easier to bear. Once it is open wide, you know that the baby is almost with you.

What if I feel I can't go on?

❝ It was painful. My midwives told me that they knew it was hard for me but that the baby was fine. That made all the difference.

❝ The three hours that transition lasted seemed endless. "When will this be over?" I kept muttering. The pain no longer seemed localised low in my abdomen. It overtook my whole body. It was huge and overwhelming.

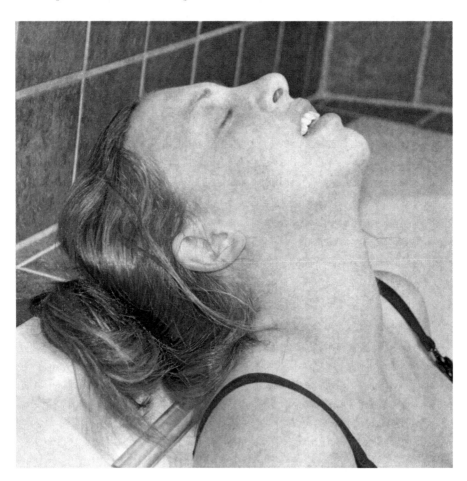

Most women feel that they can't go on and would like to postpone having the baby when they reach the end of the first stage of labour. These feelings are a sign of progress, for this is transition, the bridge between the first and second stage. You long for some rest from the storm of contractions and may get very irritable. In a long labour, or one with backache, you are likely to feel discouraged earlier than this. The words used, and the tone in which they are said, are of first importance. There is no formula that is right for every woman. But a good midwife has phrases that express her conviction that the woman can do it, in a way that is sympathetic and empowering.

I can almost hear my friend Caroline Flint murmuring encouraging words— similar to the ones I often find myself using when I am with a woman in labour:

> Good... Excellent... You're doing so well... You're beautifully relaxed... Let it happen... Let it come... Let it open you up... Surrender to it... Feel yourself opening up... Good, good, good. Well done... That's wonderful... That's marvellous... Oh, how brilliant... That's lovely... Blossom... Flourish... Open up to it... Be soft... Be giving... Surrender to it... Give, give, give... Surrender... Open, open... Good... Good, good...[13]

However tired she is, the midwife should never use these words mechanically. They express her inner awareness that the woman needs to release all tension, find her body's rhythms and open wide.

The midwife should never use words mechanically

Elizabeth Davis, midwife in San Francisco, uses such phrases as: "Keep it loose," and "Be really open and let that force move through you. Just let it be, let it down."[14]

Penny Simkin, a childbirth educator in Seattle, has what she calls the 'take charge routine' for any time in labour when a woman hits an emotional low, weeps, wants to give up, is very tense, or is in a great deal of pain. The birth partner or midwife moves in close to the mother to help her regain her inner strength. She speaks in a calm, confident voice, as she says:

❝ Breathe with me... BREATHE WITH ME... That's the way... just like that... Good... STAY WITH IT... just like that... LOOK AT ME... Stay with me... Good for you... It's going away ... Good... Good... Now just rest, that was so good.

Between contractions she may say:

❝ With the next one let me help you more. I want you to look at me the moment it starts. We will breathe together so it won't get ahead of us. OK? Good, you're doing so well. We're really moving now.[15]

Also try the suggestions on the next page, depending on the situation...

♥ If there comes a time in labour when you are discouraged, you need *change*. You can change what you are doing or change your environment.

♥ Change your position or the movements you are making.

♥ If you have background music, change the track and select a completely different rhythm or mood.

♥ Have a change of scene. Move to another room or out-of-doors. Open the window or go to the bathroom.

♥ Try changing the rhythm of your breathing. If you were tending to breathe fast, now breathe more slowly and fully. If you were breathing deeply, let your breathing speed up and allow it to 'dance' a little.

♥ Ask for a change in the kind of touch you are receiving, on a different place on your body, or a different kind of massage. Have your helpers switch over so that you are held or massaged by someone else.

♥ If other people to whom you feel close are available, ask one of them to come and be with you for a while. A fresh face often works wonders.

♥ If you have been in semi-darkness, now light a lot of candles or turn the lights up. If the room is bright, draw the curtains or dim the lights.

If there is a time when you are discouraged, you need change

♥ Change the essential oils in your massage oil, from lavender to rose, from frankincense to juniper or orange, for example.

♥ If you have had your eyes closed during contractions, open them now, and make eye contact with your birth partner or your midwife. If you have had eye contact until now, try closing your eyes and sinking down into yourself near the source of the power released deep in your body.

♥ Perhaps you have been silent during contractions. Now open up and make low sounds that go right down into your pelvis. Or, if you have been making a great deal of noise, listen to the sound of your own breathing during contractions and let each breath sound like a wave on the shingle.

♥ Freshen up. Splash your face with cold water. Get someone to brush your hair back slowly from your face. Have a bath or shower. Suck cracked ice.

♥ Pep up your energy with a glucose drink or spoonfuls of honey eaten from the pot.

What if I feel I can't control my body?

A woman who disciplines and trains her body—an athlete, swimmer, climber, dancer or regular jogger, for instance—may lose heart. She is used to mastering her body and now feels that it has let her down.

It is often claimed that dancers and horse riders have hard labours because their pelvic floor muscles are thick. But a well-exercised muscle is also a flexible muscle. It can be contracted or released at will. The problem is more likely to be that a woman who 'goes for the burn' dominates her body with stamina and courage, and can fight her labour longer. Muscular exertion will not help her in childbirth. She needs to surrender control of her muscles, and then her uterus can work for her.

It is often claimed that dancers and horse riders have hard labours because their pelvic floor muscles are thick—but a well-exercised muscle is also a flexible muscle

Ina May Gaskin, midwife at the alternative-style community, The Farm, in Tennessee, describes how she attended a cyclist who had already been in labour for 24 hours and was becoming discouraged. She says: "I was pretty sure that her problem had been that in not really 'welcoming' each rush, she was actually fighting labour in a subtle but effective way. Then I asked her what had been the longest she had ever ridden her bicycle in one day. She looked at her husband, and together they said, '120 miles,' and smiled. I said, 'Having a baby is a lot like that. It takes endurance. But you have to learn a different way of pedalling.' That seemed to make sense to her. I explained that she needed to be aware of the sensations that came with each rush and try to help open up and relax when each one came. I suggested that smooching would often aid the process. I left them alone for approximately 45 minutes, after which they called me back to check her dilation. By this time she was nearly fully dilated and was about to begin spontaneous pushing. She loved pushing and delivered her baby quite easily without a tear.[16]

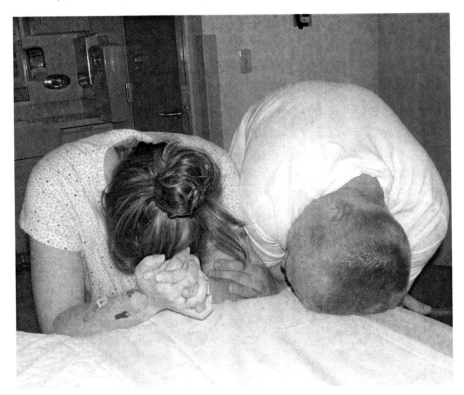

What if the midwife is worried about the fetal heart rate?

If the baby's heart rate slows or speeds up as the contraction reaches its peak, it should pick up again by about 15 seconds after the end of a contraction. If it does this, the baby is receiving sufficient oxygen.

The easiest way for your midwife to monitor this in an out-of-hospital labour is by using Doppler ultrasound—a Sonicaid held against your abdomen over the baby's heart—to listen intermittently to the heart for 30 seconds following a contraction. The Sonicaid can be used whatever your position, even under water, if it is in a polythene bag or a condom. It leaves you free to move and, because you also hear the sound, keeps you, as well as the midwife, informed.

If the fetal heart rate slows to below 100 beats per minute or increases to 160 beats and does not recover in the interval between contractions, this baby may be finding it hard-going. The problem may be that the cord has been pressed between the baby and your pelvis, and this can be solved if you change position. If you have been sitting or lying down, try standing or an all-fours position. If you are already in the second stage and have been holding your breath to push, try breathing instead, keeping your throat open. This is difficult if you are already in a pattern of breath-holding. It may help to blow out when the urge to push comes. Sometimes the baby just needs you to breathe more regularly—to keep on taking in oxygen—to have an easier birth. Your midwife will be carrying oxygen in case the baby needs a whiff after birth, and may have an oxygen mask for you to use at this point.

If, despite all your efforts, transfer to hospital is suggested, it is not failure. You have managed well up to this stage, but now need the extra help that the hospital can provide.

Once in hospital, continuous electronic fetal monitoring may be carried out, with an electrode attached to the baby's scalp. Although this provides a continuous printout, it is impossible to diagnose fetal distress accurately from it. One way of obtaining further information is to prick the baby's scalp and take a few drops of blood to be analysed. On the basis of the result you may be advised to have a forceps or vacuum extraction delivery or a caesarean section. Or the doctors may think that it is 'better to be safe than sorry' and decide, without further investigation, to deliver the baby immediately by one of these methods. This will be a shock but, after all your hard work, it may be what you want too, or you may want to discuss it further and wait a bit.

What's the best way to deal with hyperventilation?

Hyperventilation often happens at the end of the first stage, when contractions are coming at two-minute intervals

Hyperventilation is the result of breathing fast and furiously. It often happens at the end of the first stage, when contractions are coming at two-minute intervals. The woman breathes too heavily, and allows no time for the slight pauses that come naturally between inspiration and expiration and between expiration and inspiration. She feels lightheaded, giddy and nauseous, has tingling fingers, is numb around the mouth, starts to sweat, and may feel terribly panicky. Physiologically she has an increased pulse rate, a rise in blood pH (which means that the blood becomes more acidic), and blood flow to her brain decreases. A healthy baby copes well with a mother's overbreathing in labour, but a baby who is not in such good condition could be harmed by this flushing out of carbon dioxide because, when this occurs, oxygen is more firmly bound to haemoglobin and cannot be easily extracted by the cells. As a result the baby gets less oxygen.[17]

The woman breathes too heavily and allows no time for the slight pauses that come between inspiration and expiration

People often hyperventilate when under stress. Labour, especially the late first stage, is stressful. It may help if, as each contraction reaches a peak, your midwife or birth partner says: "Halfway there," or "It'll soon be over now," and uses touch to give you confidence and comfort.

You can avoid hyperventilating by keeping your shoulders and throat relaxed, by focusing on the idea of relaxing a little more with each breath out, and by letting your breathing flow rhythmically. Your helpers can breathe with you so that you do not feel so alone.

If you hyperventilate your partner can rest both hands on your shoulders and ask you to relax them and breathe more gently, with a slow sigh out. If you find this hard to do, it may help to breathe into a paper bag so that you can inhale the carbon dioxide you have exhaled. As you do this, focus on the short pause after each breath in and each breath out.

If you hyperventilate your partner can ask you to relax your shoulders and breathe more gently, with a slow sigh out

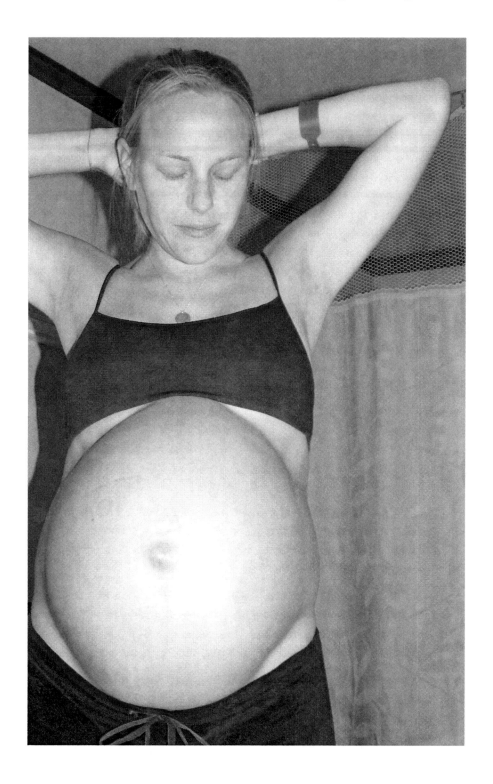

What if I get very tired?

Labour is an intense, energy-consuming activity. It may be the most strenuous work you have ever done. A woman often feels as if she is on a treadmill of contractions. The suggestions listed on pages 224-225 and 230-233 will be useful.

In some hospitals there is still a rule that a woman in labour must not eat anything, because of the danger of aspirating the contents of her stomach if she were to have a general anaesthetic. This can happen largely because gastric emptying is delayed when a woman has narcotic drugs—pethidine, for example—to relieve pain. Her only chance of being fed is through glucose and fluids via an intravenous drip. She is bound to be exhausted if she is starving, especially if she is vomiting too. She has to draw on her fat reserves for energy, with the result that she becomes dehydrated and ketones, produced by metabolisation of fat, appear in her urine.[18]

❝ After five hours I was beginning to tire of riding the pains. Anne was encouraging me all the time, saying: "Relax into it—you're doing very well—very good." She put a sponge in my mouth, I sucked on it and she wiped my face with a warm, damp flannel. She said: "Don't worry about other people. Just breathe. Keep breathing. You are doing it. You've made it. Well done!" The midwife said I was only 5cm-6cm dilated. Anne said, "You know it goes much more quickly from now on."

A woman having her baby in an out-of-hospital setting is unlikely to have analgesics that delay gastric emptying and can drink when she wishes and eat according to her appetite. So ketosis occurs less often in birth at home. But if labour is very tiring, here are some simple remedies:

- ♥ Have a drink to adjust your body's electrolyte balance. One that has been devised by American homebirth midwives is called 'Labor-Aid'.[19] You make it by mixing together 1 quart water, 1/3 cup honey, 1/3 cup lemon juice, teaspoon salt, 1/4 teaspoon baking powder, and 2 crushed calcium tablets.

- ♥ Eat something that will just slip down. You may fancy frozen yoghurt or fromage frais, some smooth porridge with honey or syrup, or a few spoonfuls of mashed mango. These will give you instant energy.

♥ Do not fight the pain. Go right into it instead. Resisting it means that you are not allowing your body to open up. A surprising release can come when we accept pain and go with it.

♥ Whatever happens during contractions, rest completely in each interval between. Drop forwards on to pillows. It is often possible to sleep for half a minute before the next contraction starts. Ask your birth partner to rest a hand on your abdomen and tell you softly when the next one is starting, so that you can tune in to it and not be taken by surprise.

♥ Remember that you are having a baby. It is easy to forget this in the thick of labour. One hospital midwife friend of mine often borrows a baby to bring to the woman in labour when she is at this stage, to remind her of what it is all about. A birth partner or a midwife says: "Come on, baby! Come on down. Come on, baby—just a little more." This may give you fresh heart.

What should I do if I want to push before I'm fully dilated?

You may have the desire to push before your cervix is fully open. Pushing hard against an incompletely dilated cervix can make it puffy and swollen so that it closes a little. This must make labour more difficult for the baby. If you want to push and are not yet 10cm dilated, you may find the following suggestions helpful:

♥ Continue breathing. Do not hold your breath. When the longing to push comes, give two quick breaths out followed by one slow breath out, so that there is a steady rhythm of pant, pant, blow, breathe in. It sometimes helps if your birth partner holds up a finger in front of your mouth, so that you can direct each blow on to it. As soon as the urge leaves you, breathe fully and easily again.

♥ If you are in an upright position, this is the time to change it and lie down on your side or be on all fours. This slightly reduces the pressure of the baby's head against your rectum and anus, so that you don't feel so desperate to push.

♥ If you have to push, do so with an open mouth and breathing out. Let your uterus do the work while you open up.

What if there's a lull at the end of the first stage?

When the baby's head is high and still above the level of the ischial spines—the bony protuberances in the pelvic cavity—there is often a pause at the very end of the first stage of labour. The uterus rests and everyone else can rest too. In hospital, during this pause, the decision is often made to set up a syntocinon drip in order to stimulate the uterus into action.

> There is often a pause... The uterus rests and everyone else rests at the same time—it's the 'rest-and-be-thankful' stage.

It is wiser to wait for descent and rotation of the head to occur and give your body a chance to prepare for the active second stage. You can use what I call the 'rest-and-be-thankful' phase to good advantage—perhaps have a shower—and come out of it refreshed and with renewed energy.

66 Everything got very quiet, with gentle contractions like ripples. I felt drowsy and dreamy. Nothing seemed to be happening. I wondered if I'd know when to push. But there was no doubt about it. After about half an hour I suddenly felt this great wave of longing and incredible rush of energy and I shouted, "Got to push!"

What about pushing?

Squatting is a good position for initiating contractions and encouraging rotation of the baby's head so that it can press against your pelvic floor muscles. When the head touches nerves in these muscles the pushing reflex is stimulated and oxytocin spurts into your bloodstream, causing strong contractions. If you start pushing simply because you are fully dilated and have been told to do so, but do not feel the spontaneous reflex, you may become exhausted with straining. You are likely to push the baby's head down unrotated, with resulting deep transverse arrest (when the baby cannot turn its head to the easiest position for delivery). In most labours this is avoidable if a woman is not urged to push too soon and if everyone waits patiently.

> Squatting is a good position for pushing

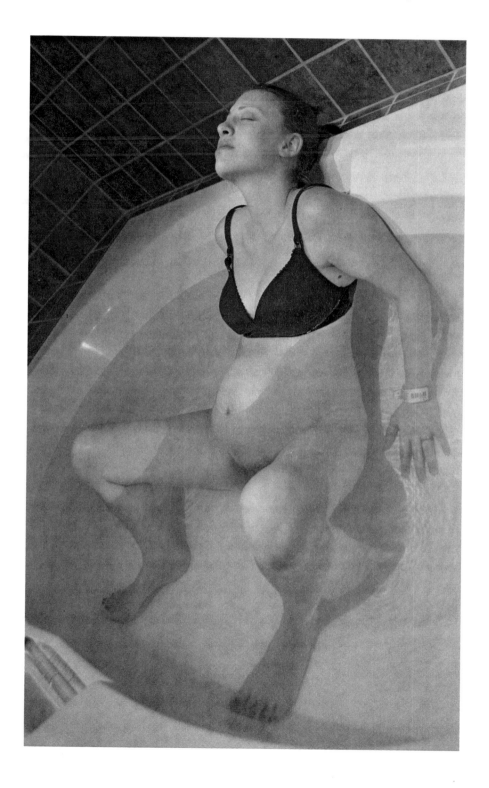

What if I don't get an urge to push?

A woman can have a baby without deliberately pushing it out. Her uterus sees to that. The energy that she gives to expulsion is only a small part—30% to 40%—of the power that is exerted by her uterus to press the baby down through the cervix, the folds of her vagina, and the spreading tissues of her perineum.

Until there is an irresistible urge to push, avoid pushing by continuing to breathe. There is no need to hold your breath deliberately at all. In this way, tissues have a chance to fan out smoothly before the ball of the baby's head eases through, with no damage to ligaments, muscles or skin.

It feels marvellous to push when you want to, and you will know exactly how to do it. When you push instinctively the second stage is a triumphant experience.

Many women and birth attendants hope to hurry the birth along by pushing before the mother's body is quite ready. This can only do harm, and it is very tiring. Commanded pushing is distressing and exhausting and often counter-productive because it makes the woman lose touch with what her body is telling her.[1] It tends to turn the second stage into a prize fight, in which she is struggling to push the baby out, blood vessels bursting in her face and eyes, and blood pressure mounting, surrounded by supporters cheering her on, regardless of her spontaneous physiological rhythms. Imagine having people encouraging you while you were making love and you will see why it is not helpful. Imposing rules on a natural physiological activity that should be spontaneous is never a good idea.

Once the baby's head touches nerves in your perineum, the Ferguson reflex is stimulated, endogenous oxytocin is released, and you want to push.[20] For some women this does not happen until the baby is just about to be born. The mother pushes once or twice and the baby slips out easily.

66 Then came the crowning. As quickly as this rush of contractions came, it stopped. I felt hot and high. I was excited. After climbing a very high mountain, I could now sit and enjoy the exhilarating view. I love this part of labour—the calm, high, ready feeling. My next contraction began and I greeted it with satisfaction. Surprised by its intensity, I let my body do it.

Sometimes the desire to push is there, but it is not strong. That's fine too. Go with your body. 'Listen' to your uterus. When the second stage has started passionately, some gentler contractions may follow in which the pushing urge is faint or non-existent. For a woman who is free to follow her uterus, the pushing rhythm may vary with different contractions. Some pushes are short and others long. Sometimes there is only one push with a contraction, at other times four or five. Even if you feel unsure about what to do, your body knows how to give birth.

What if the second stage is taking a long time?

If you want to carry on, and the baby is doing well, setting a time limit on the second stage is completely unnecessary. The second stage may be three minutes or three hours and is just right for that particular mother and baby.[21]

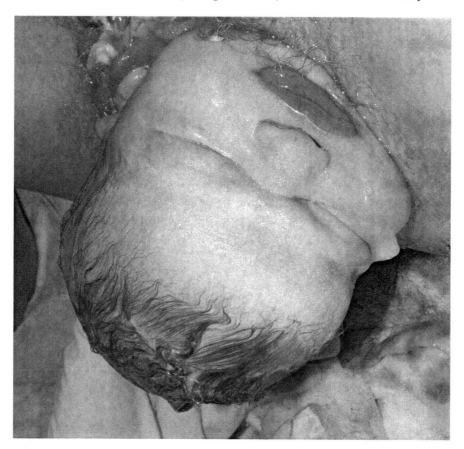

What if the baby passes meconium?

The bowels of a mature fetus contain meconium. Meconium is a sign of maturity. Thick meconium passed at the beginning of labour means that the baby has been stressed, before labour started. If the baby inhales it, there is a chance of respiratory tract infection.

Meconium is brown and sticky when fresh, green when stale. The passage of stale meconium is a sign that the baby may have been stressed in the past. If the baby is about to be born and fresh meconium is passed, your midwife or doctor will have a mucus extractor ready to suck out meconium gently—even before the baby's body is born, and before the chest has expanded to take the first breath.

It will be easier to do this if you stand with your knees bent or are on all fours, with your midwife or doctor behind you. Breathe your baby out gently, rather than pushing, and there will be time for your caregiver to suction out every bit of meconium.[22]

If you are nowhere near birth when meconium is passed, your attendants will probably suggest that you transfer to hospital so that a paediatrician can be ready to resuscitate a 'flat' baby and make sure that the airways are clear by suctioning out any contents, using an endotracheal tube if necessary. 'Flat' does not refer to a baby's shape, but to vitality at birth. A 'flat' baby is limp and floppy, and breathing is depressed.

You may feel frightened about the need for transfer. Most babies who have passed meconium during labour are perfectly all right, but having a paediatric check-up and making sure that the baby's respiratory tract is clear means that you take no chances.

A midwife:

———————————————————————————————————

66 Sometimes, while helping a mother through crowning, I feel like I'm outside a semi-trailer truck, directing the driver: "All right, bring it on a little now—hold it for a few seconds now. Okay, bring it on some more." While she holds back that tremendous force, the whole quality of her skin will change—she will relax and become more pliant and stretchy.[23]

How can I cope if the baby is coming very fast?

❝ It all happened so fast—it was all over in less than an hour. I reached hospital at 3.15pm and the midwife said I was 2cm dilated. While she was examining me, I went to 5, and the baby was born at 3.50pm. I felt steamrollered. I was shaking so much afterwards. I had to get up at 3am. and write down what had happened to get it out of my system before I could settle to sleep.

When the second stage is rapid—a precipitate second stage—and it looks as if the baby will pop out like a champagne cork, there are several things you can do to slow the pace and make the birth gentler:

♥ Adopt an all-fours position, or lie on your side, so that your midwife can 'guard' your perineum with a hand. Do not squat or stand.

♥ *Breathe* the baby out. Guide your baby down with your breathing. Avoid pushing. If you have to push, breathe again as soon as possible.

♥ Release your pelvic floor muscles and perineum, by opening your mouth, dropping your jaw, and opening your glottis. Imagine a ripe fruit with all its seeds spilling out, or even a tube of toothpaste that you have accidentally stood on, with the toothpaste oozing out, or perhaps a waterfall with a great rush of water pouring through the rocks—whatever image best helps you relax.

♥ If you want to make noises you can moo, bellow, groan, or give deep sighs. The sounds should be resonant and go right down into your pelvis. Do not scream or yelp. That will make you tighten up.

♥ Release tension and open up, letting your pelvic floor descend like a lift down to the basement, rather than holding your breath and pushing deliberately. Then your baby can glide out, without being forcibly ejected.

If you don't want to miss the birth, remember to open your eyes and reach out your arms as soon as you feel the baby slither from your body.

What happens if the baby is a surprise breech?

Occasionally labour is going well and the birth attendants see something emerging that looks like a very bald head and realise, perhaps after meconium is squeezed out, that it must be the baby's bottom. It is an undiagnosed breech.

Breech labour is like any other labour up to the point when the baby's body slips out. What may then happen is that the head gets stuck, which is why in hospitals when a breech is delivered vaginally—and many are delivered by caesarean section—a large episiotomy is done and forceps are applied to the after-coming head. Actually, most damage results from anxiety and rough handling by the person who is delivering. I have seen a doctor become anxious and pull on the baby's legs, so that the arms extended and the baby was completely stuck. A breech baby should always be delivered gently to avoid injury to the spinal cord, arms, and neck.

A breech baby should always be delivered gently to avoid injury

Left to itself, the baby's body uncurls, the uterus keeps the head flexed, and one or both legs drop out, followed by the body and then the head. In a series of 89 breech births delivered by midwives in New Jersey, USA, there was no single case of extended arms, and all the babies were fine.[24]

It is unwise to plan a breech delivery at home, because your baby may need help to breathe, and a paediatrician should be available. But if you have a surprise breech, adopt a supported, upright position, legs wide apart and knees bent, in order to give the baby's head most space and to enable gravity to help it slip through. Michel Odent says that he would "never risk a breech delivery with the mother in a dorsal or semi-seated position."[25]

The worst position for a breech delivery is lying on your back with legs raised in lithotomy stirrups, as most hospitals recommend. In that position your sacrum and coccyx are pressed up and the dimensions of your pelvic cavity and outlet are reduced. If you squat, however, you gain an extra centimetre across your pelvic cavity and two centimetres from front to back.[26]

The worst position for a breech delivery is lying on your back with your legs in lithotomy stirrups, as most hospitals recommend

Once you have adopted a half-standing, half-squatting position, leaning on your birth partner in front of you, your midwife should be positioned behind you, and simply wait and watch until the baby's body is completely born. The only intervention that may be necessary is to press gently behind the baby's knees if the feet are up over the shoulders. This will stimulate the baby to bend the knees so that they come down. When the legs are extended, they splint the spine, so that it is more difficult for the baby to take the curve of the birth canal.

As you bend your knees and go into a deep squat, holding on to your birth partner, the baby's body will slip out. The cord may slide down too, and if it is wrapped tightly around the baby, your midwife will carefully unloop it, but only very gently, or it may go into spasm. You may feel a confusing, intermittent pushing urge. Avoid pushing if you can until the head is ready to emerge. Let the baby be born by uterine activity alone. This will enable everything to open up and your tissues to spread wide. As soon as the whole body is born, drop forwards, legs still wide apart and knees bent, leaning over some furniture or your birth partner so that your back is almost horizontal. This tilts your pelvis so that the baby's nose and mouth are visible, and whoever is catching the baby can aspirate the nose and mouth with a mucus extractor before the head is fully born. A breech baby often begins to breathe once its chest is born, and may inhale mucus from your birth canal. The mucus can block the nasal passages and, although most babies are clever at sneezing out anything that is irritating, in this case aspiration is a wise precaution.

> The decision has to be made about episiotomy. Sometimes it is necessary to give the head more space.

The decision has to be made as to whether or not to perform an episiotomy. Sometimes it is necessary in order to give the head more space.

Then you will feel the crowning, with the sensation of heat and prickling that normally precede the birth, as the widest part of the baby's head passes over your perineum.

Your midwife may wrap a warm towel around the baby's body and support the head as it slides out. A breech baby may need a few whiffs of oxygen and some massage to recover from the shock of birth.

Should I have an episiotomy?

Although it is sometimes claimed that routine episiotomy rescues babies from cerebral trauma, there is no evidence for this. Randomised trials of births in which episiotomy was performed routinely or was used only when it was considered absolutely necessary reveal that no more babies have low Apgar scores or are sent to the special care nursery in the restricted episiotomy group.

A severe tear is more likely to occur when an episiotomy is performed than when a woman tears naturally. As an episiotomy heals it may be difficult to walk and sit. Many women say that it feels like sitting on jagged glass. Sometimes the episiotomy wound becomes infected, and women are more likely to have urinary incontinence and find any attempt at intercourse more painful after episiotomy than after a natural tear.[27]

Unless the baby needs to be delivered quickly, it seems sensible to decline the offer of an episiotomy.

What can we do if there is shoulder dystocia?

When a baby is vertex (head down), sometimes a big head is born and then there is delay in the delivery of the shoulders. Very rarely, the shoulders really are stuck: this is known as shoulder dystocia. The midwife can see that the baby's head is large, the cheeks are fat, and the face looks squashed. There is no sign of the neck, because it is wedged inside by the broad shoulders.

Shoulder dystocia may occur because the woman has had oxytocin stimulation of the uterus which has produced artificially strong contractions that have forced the pace, propelling a big baby along the birth canal before all the tissues have fanned out. The head shoots out and the shoulders are impacted. Women giving birth out of hospital never have labour stimulated with oxytocin, so labour tends to be slower and gentler.

Deliberate forceful pushing with prolonged breath-holding may also eject a baby's head before the tissues have fanned out sufficiently and because of this the shoulders are a tight fit. It seems better to allow labour to proceed at its own pace.

It seems better to allow labour to proceed at its own pace

The head is the largest part of the baby and like a ball that can turn on the shoulders. When the baby is nestled down, back rounded, limbs flexed, and chin tucked in, the body is like a ball, too. The head can rotate and move more or less independently of the body because of the neck, and the shoulders can rotate more or less independently of the head. If big shoulders are square on, the shoulders need to rotate so that first one can slip out, then the other.

Hospital doctors employ a range of techniques to deal with shoulder dystocia. These include pressure over the woman's pubis, a large episiotomy, fundal pressure applied over the baby's bottom, the 'Wood screw manoeuvre' that entails pushing the fingers inside and then pulling the baby out with a screwing motion, and the 'Zavanelli manoeuvre', which involves pushing the head back in again and then delivering the baby by caesarean section.[28]

If your baby's head is born and then nothing happens, move!

If your baby's head is born and then nothing happens, move! Movement often releases the shoulders. Your birth partner can help you change position. Your midwife may ask you to get on hands and knees. The antero-posterior diameter (from front to back) of your pelvis increases by as much as one or two centimetres in this position. When the next contraction comes, push hard as your helper applies gentle downwards traction to the head. The baby sometimes falls out.[29]

Or stand with your knees as wide apart as possible. Caroline Flint believes that it probably does not matter exactly how a woman moves her pelvis, "from lying down to hands and knees; from kneeling to standing up; from standing up to being on all fours—but it is important for the movement to include a tilting of the pelvis."[30] This pelvic tilt occurs automatically when you bend one knee to get up into a standing position, stride forwards, or get down on the floor.

Stand with knees as wide apart as possible and tilt your pelvis

If your baby still does not budge, your helper will reach in with two fingers and find the baby's posterior armpit, the one nearest, and either pull the shoulder forwards or pull down the arm. Ina May Gaskin says that a colleague safely delivered a 6.25kg (14lb) baby in this way. She considers that episiotomy is usually unnecessary.

What happens if the midwife suddenly finds it's twins?

The mother of twins is more likely to develop high blood pressure and pre–eclampsia, and twins are at greater risk than singleton babies, especially the second baby. The babies are often preterm and of low birth weight. One or other may lie in a difficult position. The second baby may be high, so that a loop of cord can come down before the baby's presenting part has descended. Both babies may need intensive care for the first days or weeks of their lives.

Having said this, I had my own twins at home. I was healthy, with only mild hypertension, the pregnancy went to term, the babies were known to be a good weight and were both head down, and I had an experienced midwife and a supportive partner. These are all important factors that have to be considered.

Labour was brief: they were both born in 90 minutes, one 10 minutes after the other. If I had made the journey to hospital, they would probably have been born in the car. I am glad that I weighed the risks and benefits of going to hospital and made the decision to stay at home, although I remained flexible about switching to hospital if labour was not going well, or if the babies were not in good condition. I had to make the decision without my midwife. When she arrived, she advised me to go to hospital. I asked her to examine me first. She found that the head of the first baby was already on the perineum. There was then no question of moving.

If you have undiagnosed twins or a twin labour is too fast to risk getting to hospital:

♥ Warm the room and fill hot water bottles so that the babies will not become cold. Small babies are quickly chilled.

♥ Stay calm. Breathe with a gentle expiration, as slowly as you can. You are breathing for your babies.

♥ Once in the second stage, take it as gently as possible and avoid both hyperventilating (see page 236) and prolonged breath-holding. Your first baby may cope well with these, but the second baby needs good oxygenation for a while longer.

♥ Choose any comfortable position—preferably an upright one (standing, squatting, kneeling, or half-kneeling, half-squatting). If labour is progressing very rapidly, get on all fours.

♥ When the first baby is born, put him or her to your breast. The sucking will stimulate further contractions to bring the next baby to birth.

A drug to stimulate uterine contractions (syntometrine) should never be given before the second twin is born. It results in gripping contractions of the uterus that can sometimes trap the second baby.

After the first baby is born your midwife clamps and cuts the cord, checks the lie of the second baby and listens to the fetal heart. There is space now to adjust the baby to the best position if the lie needs correcting. If labour has not started again in 15 minutes the usual practice is to rupture the membranes. However, if the firstborn is already suckling at your breast, this will stimulate further contractions that help the second baby towards birth and there may then be no need to rupture the membranes artificially.

After the birth you will sweat a lot. Even though you may feel cold and shivery, you are giving out a great deal of heat, so hold both babies against you and snuggle under the bedcovers to keep them beautifully warm.

How can we help the baby who is slow to breathe?

Babies are enormously adaptable. They can manage with very little oxygen for much longer than an adult. Some babies start to breathe as soon as their heads are born. Most take a few seconds to get going. Some start to breathe, but then breathe fitfully for as long as 20 minutes. It takes time for them to adjust. They need to be kept warm and to be touched.

When the cord is not clamped there is no rush to force breathing

When the cord is not clamped immediately, and it is pulsating, the baby is still receiving some oxygenated blood straight into her bloodstream. There need be no rush to force her to breathe.

Some babies can't breathe well because the respiratory tract is plugged with sticky mucus. When a baby is born with the mother in an upright position, any mucus drains naturally from the mouth and nose. Newborn babies often sneeze mucus out very effectively, too. If a baby needs help to breathe, the first thing to do is to make sure that the airways are clear. Your baby can be placed on his or her front with the head lower than the hips, so that mucus drains out, while you, or a helper, gently massage his or her back.

The baby's mouth can be suctioned gently too, using a mucus extractor. It is important not to stimulate the gag reflex by putting the bulb syringe down your baby's throat.

A baby who has had a difficult transition to life needs warmth. Otherwise he or she uses up energy trying to maintain body heat. Most heat loss is from the head, because it is the biggest exposed part. So your baby should be wrapped in warmed flannel blankets and his or her head covered. Sometimes a baby is completely floppy and grey and needs oxygen quickly, either mouth-to-mouth or from a bag-mask. Every midwife or doctor attending a birth should carry resuscitation equipment for the rare situation in which this is needed.

If a baby is just flickering and is starting, but not quite managing, to breathe, it helps to talk to the baby, to say, "Hello, baby," "Come on love, come on!" or "You're beautiful!" The result may be that the lungs open wider, breaths are deeper and respiration is more regular. In intensive care nurseries, where babies are being monitored very carefully, oxygen levels often rise when a baby is stroked and when the mother speaks to her baby.

Babies are more likely to have breathing problems when they are born preterm and the lungs are still immature, or when they are born in a hospital where narcotic drugs, such as pethidine or diamorphine, have been given to the mother in high doses.

In spite of the general assumption that babies are slapped on their bottoms to encourage them to breathe, the vast majority of those who are making a slow transition do not benefit from violent stimulation of this kind. If a baby seems dopey and drugged from painkillers in the mother's bloodstream, his or her feet can be tickled and, if necessary, a stimulant drug can also be injected.

In some hospitals in Eastern Europe babies are still put under a cold tap. In most hospitals elsewhere a baby who requires resuscitation is put on a special sloping shelf on his or her back, a tube is pushed down the baby's throat, he or she is mechanically ventilated, and then given oxygen by face mask. Elizabeth Davis says that she has witnessed babies whose condition worsens with this treatment, or who struggle to establish their own rhythms. "I usually find myself saying, 'Somebody touch that baby!' Or I move over and do it myself. Observation and participation has taught me that touch usually brings swift and dramatic improvement."[31]

There can be a spiritual element in helping a baby to life. Elizabeth Davis also writes of babies being tired after a long labour with a mother too exhausted to welcome a baby. "You use your heart in moments like these. 'What a gorgeous girl (or boy) you have!' Or to the sibling standing by, 'You have a sister (or brother)!' There is a tangible quality of energy that kindles life and response, pure, strong, and loving, and it's the midwife's job to work with everything she's got to initiate this at the given moment."[32]

What if I bleed heavily before I go into labour?

It is always alarming to see blood coming from your vagina during pregnancy, even if it is only a few spots. In late pregnancy you may notice slight bleeding after a vaginal examination, and sometimes after sexual intercourse. This is almost always a sign that the cervix is thin, soft and vascular, and may have started to dilate a little already. Occasionally, it is caused by a cervical polyp that has broken from its stem. This kind of bleeding stops of its own accord.

The show that often heralds labour is a blood-stained mucus plug, like the start of a period. Labour will probably begin within 24 hours after a show, although sometimes a woman goes as long as a week before contractions start. You may have several shows during labour, each heavier than the one before. This is normal.

Real bleeding is a different matter. A steady flow of blood or continual spotting can mean that the placenta is starting to peel away from the lining of the uterus (placental abruption) or that it is in front of the baby's head (placenta praevia). Let your midwife or doctor know what is happening. They will probably get you into hospital as quickly as they can, as an examination should only be done once everything has been set up for caesarean section.

Such antepartum haemorrhage may occur wherever a woman decides to have her baby and is not a risk particularly associated with out-of-hospital birth. It is much more common in women who smoke heavily. But every woman should know the symptoms just in case it happens to her.

> Antepartum haemorrhage is much more common in women who smoke heavily—but every woman should know the symptoms just in case it happens to her

How does the placenta come out?

After the baby is born your uterus continues to contract, although you may not be aware of it. The placenta cannot contract, so it peels away from the lining of the uterus, usually within half an hour of the birth, and slips down into your vagina. When this happens and the placenta is ready to be expelled, some bright red blood appears and the cord lengthens.

After the birth your uterus continues to contract

The third stage of labour, the time from the birth of the baby until the delivery of the placenta, can be conducted in two ways:

♥ Active management entails an injection of syntometrine—usually into the mother's thigh—as the baby is born, early cord clamping, and immediate removal of the placenta by cord traction.

♥ Physiological management entails allowing time for the cord to stop pulsating before clamping only the baby's end of the cord, letting blood drain into a bowl from the placental section, keeping the mother upright, and allowing her to deliver the placenta and membranes herself by pushing.

These two methods should never be mixed. To do so is a recipe for a retained placenta and postpartum haemorrhage.

Active management and physiological management should never be mixed... to do so is a recipe for a retained placenta

Until the placenta separates from the uterine wall there is no bleeding and, even though the placenta may remain in the uterus for a long time, this is not dangerous. Your midwife may press in above your pubic bone and push upwards towards your navel to see if the cord moves up as the uterus is tipped upwards. If it does, the placenta is still attached and no one should pull on the cord, or it may cause bleeding. In hospitals, sometimes an energetic attempt to complete the third stage results in the cord breaking. I have also known of women who have had the uterus pulled right down in this way.

Physiological management entails allowing time for the cord to stop pulsating before clamping, keeping the mother upright and allowing her to deliver the placenta herself by pushing

The partner of a woman who gave birth without assistance phoned me to announce a happy birth three hours before and asked, "When should we expect the placenta?" I advised him to call a midwife, which he declined to do because the local health authority had refused to allow them a home birth. So I suggested that he help his wife into an upright position and, if the placenta did not fall out, that she should remain kneeling and put her lips around the stem of a bottle and give a long blow into it. She did this and the placenta dropped out. It is a traditional practice in South America to free a retained placenta. As air is exhaled, the abdominal press comes into play so that the mother's abdominal muscles press on her fundus and propel the placenta down. This is far safer than heaving the uterus around manually or tugging on the cord.

Kneeling upright and blowing into a bottle is a traditional practice in South America to free a retained placenta

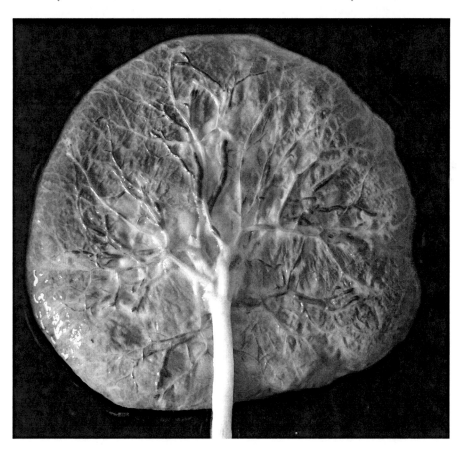

What if there's too much bleeding in the third stage?

Occasionally a placenta does not peel away completely and blood seeps from gaping sinuses in the muscle wall of the uterus. This is postpartum haemorrhage. It is more likely to occur after the uterus has been stretched with a twin pregnancy or with excess amniotic fluid, when a woman has haemorrhaged with a previous birth, following a difficult labour, or in a case where there has been 'fundus fiddling' by an anxious attendant. Elizabeth Davis says: "Left to itself the uterus will clamp down uniformly and will sheer off the placenta in one smooth sweep. But if poked and prodded it may only release in certain sections."[33]

With postpartum haemorrhage the mother's blood pressure drops. Especially in poor countries many women are anaemic and cannot afford a heavy blood loss. Elizabeth Davis recommends that a woman in poor health in late pregnancy should have supplementary B vitamins (100mg daily), plenty of protein- and iron-rich foods, and alfalfa tablets. Alfalfa is rich in Vitamin K which facilitates the clotting of blood.[34]

The first thing for the midwife to do if there are signs of haemorrhage is to give an intravenous injection of syntometrine and, if necessary, press the uterus firmly between two hands. A woman bleeds only if her uterus is soft and spongy and does not contract. It should be firm to the touch. If it is not, someone should massage it to stimulate it to contract. You can do this yourself, pressing in as if you are squeezing meringue mixture through an icing nozzle. Nipple stimulation, either from the baby breastfeeding, or done manually, also keeps the uterus firm. Once the uterus is firm and contracting, adopt a squatting or all-fours position, and the placenta should be delivered by steady, controlled cord traction with you in this position.

When the placenta is delivered, your midwife will check your pulse and blood pressure and may ask you to continue massaging your uterus to keep it well-contracted. She will stay with you for the next two hours or so.

Nowadays a healthy woman with high haemoglobin in pregnancy can cope with blood loss without having reduced haemoglobin afterwards. All the same, after a bleed it is sensible to take supplementary iron and to eat iron-rich foods such as chocolate, eggs, molasses, dried fruits, watercress, and other green leafy vegetables. A blood test will be done a few days later to check your haemoglobin level.

Labour at home and in birth centres does not suffer aggressive intervention so emergencies are extremely rare events

The sudden, dramatic dash to hospital, sirens screaming; the grey and floppy baby who is barely breathing; the woman haemorrhaging massively— these fears are at the back of all our minds. But, because labour at home and in birth centres does not suffer the aggressive intervention to which many hospital labours are subjected, they are extremely rare events.

There is no single ideal birth. There is instead the birth you have, the experience that is uniquely yours. With the support of friends who are sensitive to your needs, quick to respond to your wishes and nurture you, and who above all believe in you and your ability to give birth, childbirth can be an adventure in physical sensation and intense emotion, a journey of discovery of your own inner power that is exhilarating, sensuous and satisfying.

Childbirth can be an adventure in physical sensation and intense emotion, a journey of discovery of your own inner power that is exhilarating, sensuous and satisfying

A carefully planned and lovingly conducted home birth, in which the rhythms of nature are respected by a midwife with knowledge and understanding to support the spontaneous unfolding of life, is the safest kind of birth there is.

> 66 This delivery was so much exactly what a birth should be like, and it made such a strong impression and has given me such an 'easy', confident person of a baby, that I shall always be grateful.... It wasn't an earth-shattering experience but almost the opposite—a simple, straightforward event that happened naturally as part of the rhythm of the day.

A carefully planned and lovingly conducted home birth, in which the rhythms of nature are respected by a midwife with knowledge and understanding to support the spontaneous unfolding of life, is the safest kind of birth there is

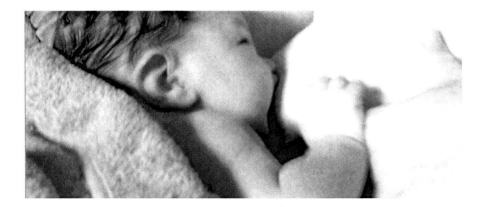

Enjoying your babymoon

The time immediately following birth is precious. It should never deteriorate to being merely a sequel to delivery, an interval for postpartum recovery, or the kind of 'bonding' time in which you feel you must fall in love with the baby fast, or you are being an inadequate mother. In birth we have the opportunity ourselves to be reborn, to see the world with new clarity, and to experience life with an intensity that may otherwise be forgotten. A child is born and for a moment the wheeling planets seem to stop in their tracks as past, present and future meet. This sense of the miraculous, of incarnation and transcendence, often floods in wherever a baby is born. But when a woman is in her own space, when a couple feel at home in the environment in which they meet this new life, there is a special radiance. Being in a place that you control yourselves means that you need not conform to any standards, be self-consciously on your best behaviour, or worry about what other people are thinking of you. Instead, you are free to focus entirely on the baby.

PLANNING YOUR BABYMOON

❝ Our neighbours had noticed the comings and goings of the midwives' cars, so my father put up a notice in the window on pink card announcing Grace's arrival. The whole episode became a social event rather than a medical occasion. We plied the midwives with champagne, forgetting they'd missed their lunch, and sent them reeling on their way about 6 o'clock.

❝ It was well after 2 o'clock on Christmas morning. It was slightly snowing outside and Naomi was peacefully nursing at my breast. We celebrated for another couple of hours before everybody left to get ready for their Christmas celebrations at home.

The babymoon is the old 'confinement' in contemporary idiom, adapted to the needs of a woman who, instead of having an extended family, experiences the deepest closeness with her sexual partner. It is a special time in the growth of love and for many couples has a significance greater than that of the honeymoon, with consequences that may be long-lasting.

The idea of a babymoon is simply that the couple create a setting in which they are intimately alone with their baby, and can get to know him or her without the intrusion of the usual responsibilities and social contacts

The idea is simply that the couple create a setting in which they are intimately alone with their baby and can get to know him or her without the intrusion of the usual responsibilities and social contacts. Your midwife calls in each day at first, to check on you and the baby, but otherwise you limit other people to a set visiting time, so that your intimacy is not invaded. All the baby-admiring and cuddling and cups of tea and sips of champagne can take place with friends and relatives sitting on and around the bed. At other times you have a note on the door that reads: 'Please do not disturb. Mother and baby resting.'

Unless you already have a child and would welcome someone close to you who can give extra attention to the other child while you get to know your baby, this might mean putting off having your mother to stay, for example, till the end of this week or 10 days, or however long you want the babymoon to last. It also entails careful planning ahead so that your partner can take time off work and you have food in store. If you have a freezer, you can shop and cook well ahead of time. Even if you don't, ensure that the cupboards are full. Before you start labour, buy plenty of fruit juices and other drinks, since breastfeeding makes you thirsty.

Your partner will have to be chef, housekeeper and butler

Your partner will have to be chef, housekeeper and butler, unless you are going to rely entirely on takeaway meals and let the dirty dishes pile up. The phone is bound to ring a lot. Work out together how you want to deal with that. As well as time to cuddle, you will want time to sleep.

LYING IN

Traditionally women have always had a 'lying in' time, a period of seclusion in which they could concentrate on the new baby and be cared for by other women. Although in situations of extreme poverty, war or famine it is impossible to ensure this, it remains the ritual ideal in many cultures and is a powerful functional bond in women's domestic culture.[1] The 40 days after birth are a time when the new mother is exempt from at least some of her usual tasks and she receives special consideration, nourishing foods and loving support from other women of the household, as she passes over the bridge into motherhood. Many of these women stay in the new mother's home for days or weeks afterwards.[2]

      ❝ This is when birth at home is so wonderful. You can sleep if and when you want, have the light on to look at your baby when you want, eat and drink when you want. Your husband and children are with you, and everybody can feel uninhibited in greeting and responding to the new baby at their own pace.

During the earliest part of this period you are in an enclosed space, sometimes a darkened room, and access to outsiders is severely restricted. For you are in a marginal social and spiritual state, and you and the baby are considered to be especially vulnerable and tender.

Within traditional Judaic culture the new mother was cared for entirely by other women for the first 30 days after birth. They built a fire by her and this was fed even on the Sabbath, when such work was normally forbidden, and she was plied with sugary teas and nourishing food.

Usually the time of intensive loving care is shorter than this. In Fiji, for example, the new mother is tended by both of the grandmothers with two young women from her own kin group and two from the father's until the 10th day. In all traditional cultures there are nurturing women to help care for the new baby, take over household tasks, such as cleaning and washing, and perhaps massage both mother and baby. They pride themselves on producing especially sustaining foods. In parts of India, for example, they prepare a drink of sweet coconut milk mixed with dill seed, which is thought to give the mother strength.

In today's industrial society women are often expected to take over cooking and cleaning and caring for their husbands and other children, and to demonstrate that they have 'got their figures back' within a few weeks, and sometimes mere days, after birth. They want to return to 'normal', as if nothing has happened. It is all supposed to take place without a second thought, and with tremendous joie de vivre. Yet if a new mother is to be able to nurture her child, she herself needs to be nurtured. Most women need space and time and cherishing from those closest to them, to make the major adjustment to motherhood, and the focus should be on neither recovery nor return, but rather on transformation.

If you are having your baby at home, or if you are returning home soon after the birth—the usual arrangement if you have your baby in a birth centre—my suggestion is that you may enjoy postpartum 'nesting' in a king-sized bed. The whole focus of the home switches to the bed with its new life. It is as if, for a short space, your bed becomes the household shrine.

My suggestion is that you enjoy postpartum 'nesting' in a king-sized bed. It's as if your bed becomes the household shrine.

WELCOMING YOUR BABY

> ❝ I couldn't help grieving a little. It felt so magical to have her inside me. I had a feeling of emptiness when she was born. She was beautiful, but different from how I had imagined.

When a woman first meets her baby, she says goodbye to the fantasy baby inside her and greets the real one in her arms. This can be a difficult transition for a woman who had a clear idea that the baby was of one sex and it turns out to be the other, or who was sure that the baby would be perfectly formed and a handicap is revealed, or who expected that the baby would look like her or her partner, or be smaller or larger or more attractive than it actually is. A woman strives to find continuity of experience between the baby inside and the baby outside her body. It is not just that she needs time to come to terms with this reality. She may also need a sanctuary in which she can experience safely a range of conflicting emotions. A hospital is a difficult place in which to do this, with all its comings and goings, the routines of a large institution and the social isolation from those closest to her that is often imposed on the new mother while she remains a 'patient'.

> ❝ I knew instantly that she was mine. But there was an odd detachment too. It was as if there were two babies and the baby inside me was retreating from me while Imogen was coming towards me. Part of me mourned that dark, mysterious baby inside me. At the same time I looked at Imogen and thought, "We've arrived! Here is my family." Now this house is full of children, and that's how I want it to be.

For many women who have their babies in hospital bonding is delayed and hindered, or sometimes never gets going, until after they are home, and occasionally not even then.

For many women who have their babies in hospital bonding is delayed and hindered, or sometimes never gets going until later

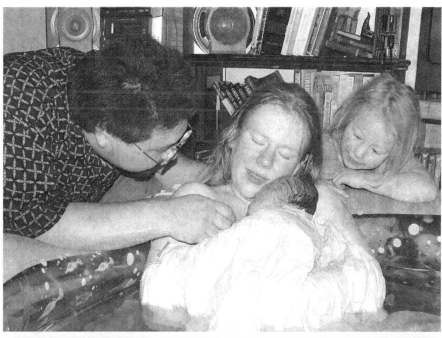

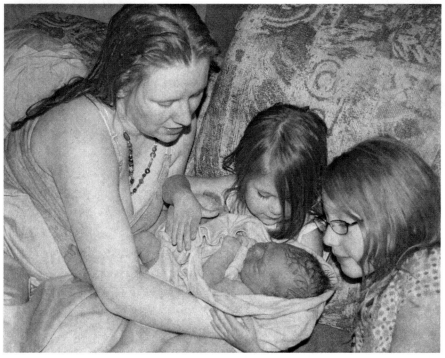

Only in a warm, loving and intimate environment can a woman feel secure in expressing her real emotions

New mothers tell of the frustration, demoralisation and depression at feeling caught up in an alien and threatening system that they are powerless to influence in any way, either for themselves or for their babies. They say such things as: "The nurses were liable to take the babies away with no explanation and were surprised when asked what they were about to do"; "I felt like one of the cogs in a machine, not a person at all"; and "The mothers seemed to be there for them, and not the other way round."

Hospital staff may consider that the new mother's prime need is for rest and want to ensure that each woman has uninterrupted sleep at night, and rest times during the day, apart from her baby. In some hospitals, for example, babies born at night tend to be sent to the nursery even though they are perfectly all right, because it is the easiest thing to do, and it avoids disturbing other mothers.

One result of awareness of the importance of bonding and of failure to bond being viewed as a cause of child abuse is that in some hospitals nurses are on the lookout for potential child abusers. Sometimes mothers are acutely aware that they are under critical observation to reveal if they are responding appropriately to their babies. One woman, whose baby suffered from facial palsy, said, "They thought I was in danger of rejecting the baby," and she felt that they thrust him at her. Every time she went to the special care baby unit she felt that she had to put on a performance, and so began to avoid visiting it. The staff's enthusiasm to promote bonding actually made it more difficult for this woman to accept her baby.

Only in a warm, loving and intimate environment can a woman feel secure in expressing her real emotions. Mothering grows from genuine feelings and bears no resemblance to the magazine image of a glamorous mother in a frilly negligee proudly cradling her new baby. When a woman becomes a mother, she may be swept along as if on a rollercoaster of fierce, passionate and often conflicting emotions. Her identity as the mother of this particular child is forged not only through pleasure in her baby, but also through the anxiety, pain and other negative feelings which stem naturally from the 'primary maternal preoccupation' that is a normal accompaniment to falling in love with a baby.[3]

To carry a child in your body, to plan ahead, to make choices between alternatives, to give birth and hold your baby in your arms is an experience that can bring with it profound emotional commitment, deep acceptance of responsibility and a maturing of personality. It is not a medical event. It is a major life transition.

When you greet your baby on your own territory, those who help you come as guests, not guardians of medical space. The whole obstetric system is designed to control women, to render them passive and to screen, treat and regulate their reproductive functions for their own good. But in your space there are no rules to be obeyed, no standards to which you must conform. You are free to be yourself.

Lying together in bed with your baby, you both have time to explore the astonishing reality of this new little being

Lying together in bed with your baby, you and your partner both have extended time to explore the astonishing reality and the wonder of this new little being. You relive the experience of birth, learn how to respond to his signals and can start breastfeeding at your own pace and in your own way. Your older children may enjoy cuddling in with you for some of the time, and at other times will need a loving person who can focus on their needs and enable you to have this special time with your baby.

You feel your baby's plump firmness in your arms, stroke the down on the head and see bright eyes gazing up at you. There is an excitement about breastfeeding that is going well. It is partly the conviction that your body is working well and you can both give life and sustain it, partly the sensual physical contact, pleasurable holding and the surge of the milk flow, and partly the preverbal conversation with this small human being in your arms, as you get to know a wide-eyed creature for whom the whole world is new, who comes to you out of its raw, elemental being and turns to you in trust.

" I felt my whole body and consciousness expand and fill with pleasure. At that moment I felt that I had been the agent of a miracle, had brought about a revelation not of a truth, but of a life, and with it immense humility and gratitude.

You will both become aware of your baby's rhythms, the cycles of sleep and waking, the times when he is alert, other times when he is fretful or drowsy, and the highpoints of his life, when he wakes hungry and discovers the firm sweetness of his mother's breasts and sucks avidly until he falls asleep, replete and utterly satisfied. You will enjoy 'conversations' with your baby when he is in an awake and alert state. A baby is not merely at the receiving end of stimuli. He can communicate with you using his attention, the steady gaze of his eyes, his restlessness, or the glazed expression that comes on his face before he falls asleep at last. Parents don't need code books to understand this. All they require is unhurried time with their baby in an environment where they can act with spontaneity and are not inhibited by anybody else's expectations or theories. It is an environment that hospitals find very difficult to provide. But it exists already. It is home.

ADJUSTING EMOTIONALLY

The change from woman to mother occurs as if by grace, by enchantment... but it is also fraught with pain

There is emotional work to be done too. The change from woman to mother occurs as if by grace, by enchantment, but it is also fraught with pain. When you have a baby your view of the world changes. You see people, and other people's children, with new eyes. You become more vulnerable, more touched by suffering, more sensitively aware of need. You may weep more readily, be distressed by items on news programmes, feel bonded not only with your baby, but with all human beings, all living things, in a different way. Your whole relationship with time changes and is moulded around your child's need of you. You often feel that time stretches out endlessly like a long ribbon with no end in sight. However it is, you cannot go on as before. Life has a new shape.

You often feel that time stretches out endlessly like a long ribbon with no end in sight. However it is, you cannot go on as before. Life has a new shape.

The transformation of woman to mother often has to occur in isolation from that of man to father and, as a result, is qualitatively entirely different. After they have a child, many couples find that they each speak a different language and have widely divergent concerns. The mother is child-focused. The father is work-focused. This often happens even when the woman has a career, and up until now has had work at the centre of her life. A man may see a new baby as a possession, but for a woman the child is her flesh. Thus her identity is changed fundamentally, while his is not. You both need a space in your lives to pass through the transformation into being parents, to adjust together to the nakedness of feelings, the new fluidity of time and the new centre to your lives.

66 My other two children saw her within minutes. For them birth is a normal process which can happen in the next bedroom, not a dark technological mystery.

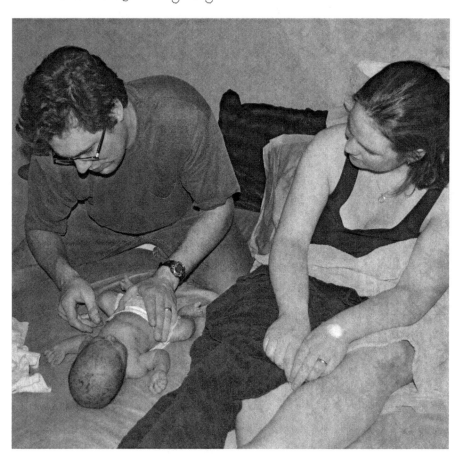

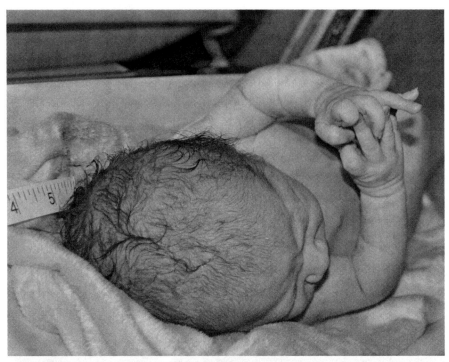

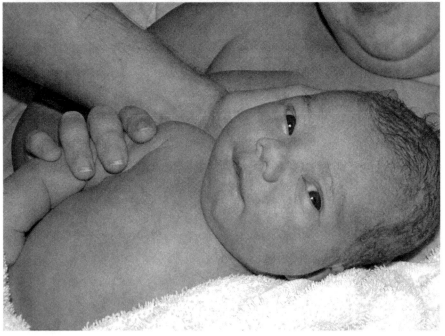

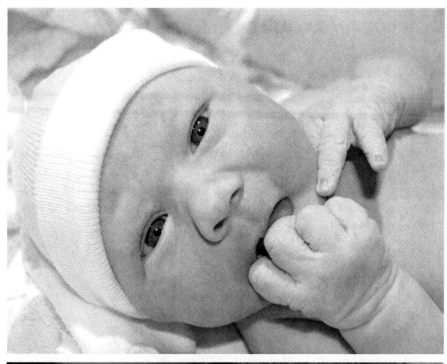

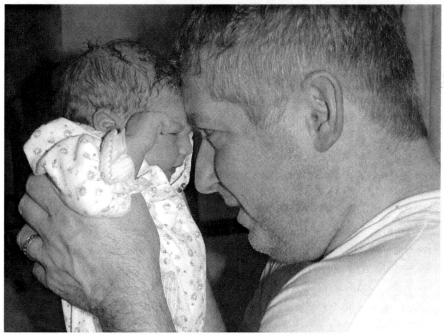

CONSIDERING YOUR OTHER CHILDREN

If you already have a child, this oasis in time is one that nurtures your older child too. She also has to pass through a transformation, from special and only one to older sister, from baby to child. This process of growth cannot be rushed. She, too, needs time and a sanctuary. If your bed is big enough, she can cuddle up with you and the new baby, assured of your love for her, able to get to know the baby in her own way. Keep special playthings and story books close by, and have some favourite snacks handy. She won't want to stay with you long, but will bounce off to play, make things, have an adventure. Your partner will be kept busy coping with your older child's needs as well as yours. This kind of babymoon has a different flavour!

An older sister:

66 It was good that my mum had the baby in the holidays because I was so excited that I did not get to sleep until 3 o'clock in the morning. For a whole week we had dinner in my mum's room with champagne. Like a picnic to celebrate.

STARTING TO BREASTFEED

Women can breastfeed against amazing odds. I have been in hospitals in Russia where mothers are not handed their babies until four hours or longer after birth, by which time nurses have already swaddled them, and where women must have their fingers painted with iodine before they can touch their babies. Yet they breastfeed successfully—because they know they can, and the alternative of artificial feeding is not readily available.

Breastfeeding in hospital

The average hospital environment provides the worst possible start for breastfeeding. In spite of all the lip service paid to breastfeeding in Britain, for example, in 30% of big hospitals with consultant units women still could not as a matter of course put their babies to the breast at birth. In 40% of hospitals babies did not 'room in' with their mothers all the time, and 16% of hospitals allowed babies to be with their mothers only in the daytime.[4]

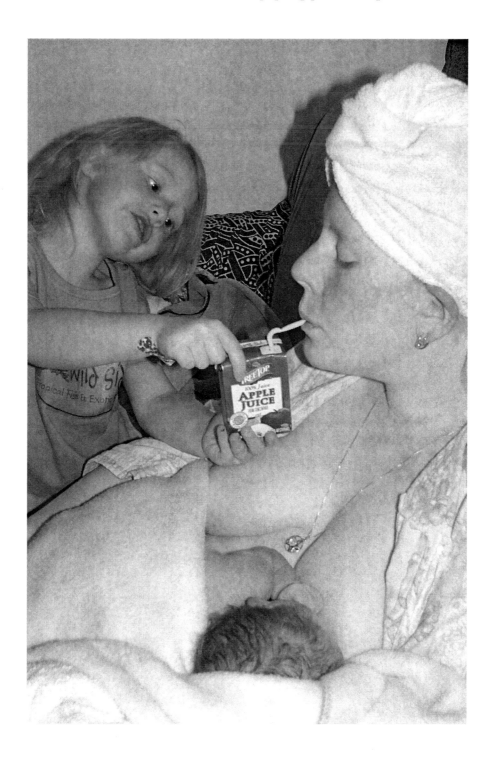

Babies are separated from their mothers 'so that you can rest', "so that the baby isn't overstimulated," "so as not to disturb the other mothers," "so that we can keep an eye on him", "because there is a rule that the baby must be in the nursery for the first two nights, and your milk hasn't come in, so there is no point in having him with you" or "because the baby is slightly jaundiced and needs phototherapy."

Hospitals are noisy places and in some sedatives are given routinely at night to all mothers, including those who are breastfeeding. One woman commented: "Going without a sleeping tablet seems to be regarded as a perversion." Crying babies are often whisked away to the nursery, may be given formula by nurses who try to keep the ward peaceful, and who may also enjoy the chance to feed and look after the babies.

Only 30% of hospitals give no additional fluids to breastfed babies: 25% offer water if they think the baby needs it, 7% offer it routinely, and 38% give the babies glucose solution and/or artificial milk.[5]

Women are the target of a great deal of conflicting advice from different caregivers too. They often feel they have to show that they are following the advice given by whoever is watching them at the time and, as a result, become bewildered and disheartened. They sometimes comment that although usually capable and self-assured, they seemed especially vulnerable in hospital and were surprised at how easily they felt put down or humiliated.

There is general approval of 'demand feeding' in many hospitals. Yet even within the same hospital, there may be different interpretations of what this actually is. Many nurses see it as feeding whenever the baby cries, but not more often than every two hours or less often than every five hours. In some hospitals mothers are encouraged to follow their babies' lead but must fill in forms indicating when they have fed. They often find it difficult to do this in a relaxed and spontaneous way because, as one said, "I felt inhibited about owning up to each nibble of colostrum." As a result they 'cheat' on the charts and give the impression that the baby is suckling less often than is the case.[6]

A father:

66 Ally was very tired after the birth but, because she was at home, she could rest. If she had been forced to adapt to a hospital routine, I think she would have been utterly exhausted.

Regulations to keep other staff members happy, including doctors, ward cleaners and caterers, or to present the ward as an orderly, well managed place to visitors, sometimes restrict feeding times to certain hours. So mothers may be told that they must not feed at mealtimes, during ward cleaning, at rest times, during the physiotherapy exercise session, during doctors' ward rounds, when they should be having a bath, and at visiting times. As one woman said, "The hospital seemed to treat babies' feeding times as a necessary evil interrupting hospital routine." As a result babies cry a lot. An Asian mother in a London hospital, wondering at the strange way in which Europeans seem to treat their babies, asked, "Why do the English punish their babies?"

> An Asian mother asked: "Why do you punish your babies?"

The most usual reasons that are cited for giving up breastfeeding are 'insufficient milk', that the baby 'rejected the breast' or 'failed to latch on', and 'sore nipples'.[7]

Some nurses approve of breastfeeding if it comes easily, but expect mothers to switch to artificial feeding if there are problems, and to stay relaxed about it. They often give tireless devotion, sitting with women to help them establish breastfeeding but some do not understand the skills of breastfeeding and the art of encouraging a baby to latch on.

They are also concerned that emphasis on breastfeeding makes those mothers who are advised to feed artificially feel that they are failures, and seem to hope for a slightly detached attitude in the mother. One woman who resisted the suggestion that her baby should be artificially fed wrote, "The nurse said she had expected trouble with me because I was 'one of those mothers who are determined to breastfeed, come what may'."

It is not surprising that in Britain, in one study, 19% of first-time mothers and 15% of all mothers have stopped breastfeeding even before they leave hospital, and that by the end of the sixth week after birth only 38% are still breastfeeding, and at four months only 26%.[8] Nearly half of all breastfed babies have artificial milk supplements within their first week of life. By the end of the second week 28% of those babies who had supplementary feeds are fed artificially, compared with only 8% of those who had no supplementary feeds.

> It's not surprising that so many mothers in Britain stop breastfeeding before they leave hospital

❝ I was given Hilary almost immediately while they dealt with the placenta. She suckled straight away. She was beautiful. When everyone had left and she had been put in her crib, she wouldn't settle, so I lifted her out and I lay nursing her for the rest of the night. Neither Duncan nor I had experienced such complete happiness ever before.

Neither of us had experienced such complete happiness before

Your own space for breastfeeding

The joy of starting breastfeeding in your own environment is that you do not have to put on a demonstration to anyone or prove that you can do it successfully. Instead, it is a secret and delightful conspiracy between you and the baby. Breastfeeding is a natural element in your developing relationship that is exciting and satisfying for you both, an adventure in sensation and touch, and in the gradual unfolding of personality of this new human being and this new mother. Breastfeeding is a way of communicating, a way of loving. Because this is so, it is never merely a matter of technique.

The joy of starting breastfeeding in your own environment is that you do not have to put on a demonstration to anyone or prove that you can do it successfully

There may be pain mixed strangely with the tenderness and desire. As your baby's sucking stimulates contractions of the uterus, helping it to return almost to its pre-pregnant size and shape, your breasts become full, heavy and swollen. When the baby latches on, you experience the urgency of the milk ejection reflex and your breasts become flushed and hot.

When you are in your own intimate place, a place that you have created, you realise that breastfeeding is not just a matter of what a woman does with her breasts, but rather of her sense of positive identity as a woman and a mother and that when she breastfeeds an intense flow of energy surges through her whole body.

When you are in your own intimate space you realise that breastfeeding is part of your identity as a woman, as a mother

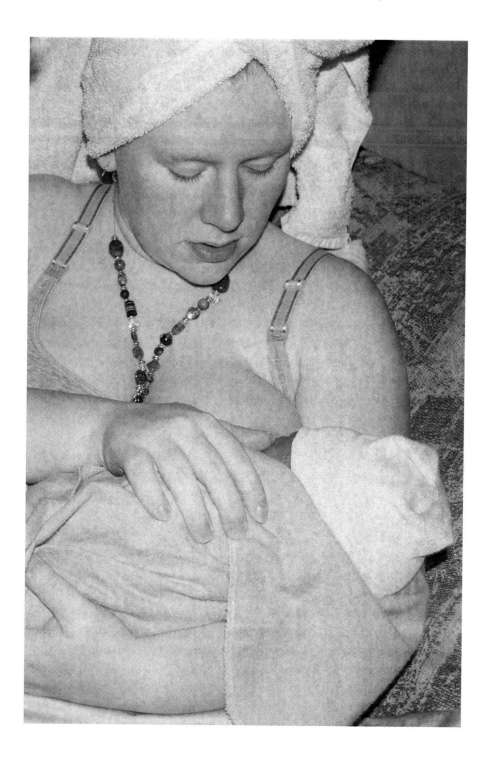

Even after your babymoon has finished, you can keep the same closeness if you have 'night nesting'. By this I mean that you have your baby sleeping in bed with you or close beside, instead of in a cot. Traditionally, mothers have always slept with their babies and still do so in many cultures, even in the highly evolved industrial society of Japan. In contrast, Western emphasis on children's development of autonomy—being independent and achieving—dictates that a baby should be in his or her own cot, in his or her own room, and should not disrupt adult activities.

NIGHT NESTING

When you have your baby within arms reach, the physical closeness, the sounds of your breathing and beating heart, and the warmth of your body are comforting for your baby, and having the baby beside you to touch and to gaze at when you wish is reassuring for you. However busy and rushed you are during the day, night nesting ensures undisturbed time with your baby. You can breastfeed without really waking and, provided that the baby is not sandwiched between you, snuggle down with your baby falling asleep again still on your breast.

This is not dangerous. Healthy newborns move their heads away if their noses are obstructed and are in no danger of being 'overlaid', although it is wise not to have a baby in bed if either you or your partner has been drinking heavily or has taken drugs that reduce awareness. A really large bed with a firm mattress makes this arrangement more comfortable for all of you. However, there is also an advantage in accustoming the baby to sleeping separately sometimes too, so that later on you do not always have to go to bed every time you want your child to settle down.

If you are going back to work again soon after the birth, night nesting and breastfeeding whenever your baby wants to stimulates milk production, and means that you can continue breastfeeding even if your baby is being cared for by someone else for the major part of the day. You may have such a good milk supply that you need to express milk while you are at work lest you become engorged. You can do this simply with a small, portable electric pump, or even by hand if you are adept at it. Then you can store this milk in a refrigerator so that someone else can give it to the baby in a bottle.[9]

All over the world, in widely varying cultures, women breastfeed while at the same time working in and outside their homes, labouring in the fields, cracking stones to make roads, washing the family's clothing in the river, or gathering berries and other foods in the bush. It is part of a busy life in which the baby is breastfed wherever the mother happens to be, and the baby may suck on and off through the hours of darkness. This is a pattern of breastfeeding which works well, and one that women in industrial societies are now rediscovering for themselves.

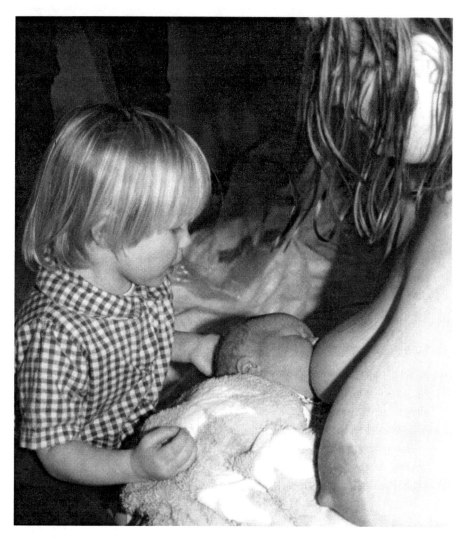

" Demand feeding was easy as I had the baby in bed with me.

Breastfeeding Q&A:

Q: Why is breastfeeding important for me?

A: In addition to the advantages for the baby, breastfeeding is not just a matter of what you do with your breasts, but your sense of positive identity as a woman and a mother. An intense flow of energy surges through your whole body. There is evidence that it reduces the risk of breast cancer, too.

Q: Is there an advantage in beginning breastfeeding at home?

A: Yes. It is usually easier to establish breastfeeding at home. The joy of starting to breastfeed in your own environment is that you do not have to put on a demonstration or prove to your carers that you can do it successfully. Instead, it is a secret and delightful conspiracy between you and the baby.

Q: Will breastfeeding help me bond with my baby?

A: Yes. Breastfeeding is a natural element in your developing relationship that is exciting and satisfying for you both, an adventure in sensation and touch and the gradual unfolding personality of this new human being. Because this is so, it is never merely a matter of technique. It is a way of communicating and loving.

Q: Does breastfeeding hurt?

A: At first there may be pain mixed strangely with tenderness and desire. Your baby's sucking stimulates contractions of the uterus, helping it return almost to its pre-pregnancy size and shape. Your breasts become full, heavy, swollen and tender. When the baby latches on, you feel the urgency of the milk ejection reflex and your breasts get flushed, hot and tingling. Make sure that the baby is well latched on, with a good mouthful of breast, or your nipples will become sore and painful.

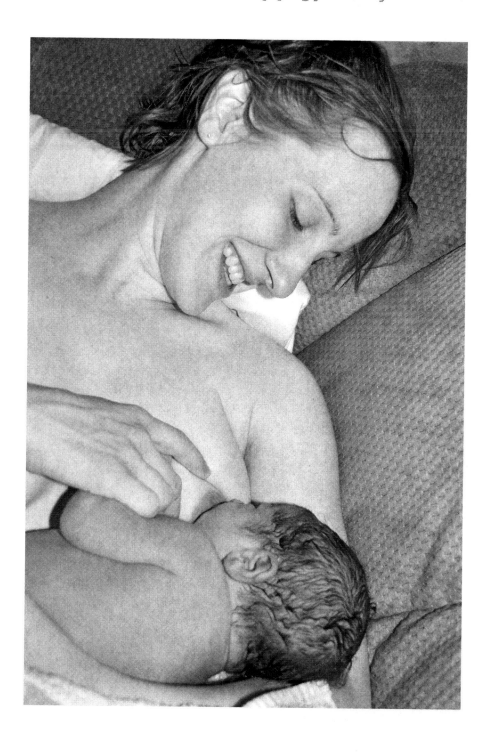

DEALING WITH DIFFICULT EMOTIONS

Nobody knows how many women are unhappy after childbirth. In Western countries one in 10 receives medical treatment for depression.[10]

Nobody knows how many women are unhappy after childbirth.
A great many women do not realise they are depressed.

Almost half of those treated are still depressed a year later. But this is just the tip of the iceberg. A great many women do not realise that they are depressed, and many of those who do have no help in dealing with their depression. New mothers often seek advice about breastfeeding difficulties, for example, yet are really asking for help with their own inturned anger and feelings of helplessness and worthlessness. Statistics of clinical depression do not include these distressed women.

Postnatal depression

Postnatal depression is often envisaged as a kind of mental fog that seeps out of a woman's bloodstream and reproductive organs. According to this view, nothing can be done to prevent it and when it happens women are treated as if they are sick. They may be prescribed mood-changing drugs and be told that ultimately the cure lies within themselves. But, in fact, depression has specific social causes and there may be many things in a woman's life that contribute to it.

Depression after the birth of a baby is less to do with the hormonal disturbance to which it is often attributed than to all the pressures on a woman to conform to the pattern of a happy new mother, to the socio-economic stresses on women who are living in poverty,[11] and, very often, to the experience of being disempowered during childbirth. My own research reveals that the institutional violence typical of care in many hospitals results in the depersonalisation and disabling of women. As a result, some new mothers are left trying to cope with feelings that are very similar to those a woman experiences after being raped, and which often persist weeks, months and even years later.[12]

In fact, depression has specific social causes and
there may be many things in a woman's life that contribute to it

There is debate among psychologists and sociologists as to whether obstetric intervention in childbirth is associated with depression. Some research suggests that the more obstetric intervention takes place, the more women suffer from depression.[13] Certainly women are more likely to be depressed after a caesarean section.[14]

A woman's sense of control is important

Women who feel that they were denied any control over what was done to them in childbirth are at greater risk of being unhappy in the week following birth than those who feel that they were in control.[15] This is different from depression, although it may turn into depression. It is post-traumatic stress disorder (PTSD), emotional distress which men, too, may suffer after traumatic events in which they were powerless.[16] It is not so much whether there is intervention, but a woman's sense of control or loss of control over what is being done to her, that is important. This may be why women who have planned caesarean sections are less likely to suffer postnatal depression than those who have unplanned caesarean sections, when the decision is made once labour has started, often over their heads and over their supine bodies.[17]

Women who have PTSD after a first baby sometimes decide to have the next birth at home because they are convinced that the hospital environment was in large measure responsible for their later emotional distress. There is mounting evidence that they are right and that a woman's feelings of wellbeing are enhanced when she is able to give birth in an environment that she herself controls. When you give birth in an environment of your own making you are more likely to experience postnatal euphoria than postnatal depression, anxiety or panic.

I am not claiming that if you have your baby at home you will never feel unhappy or unable to cope. But pervading anxiety, panic attacks, loss of confidence, feelings of worthlessness and an uneasy sense that the baby does not really belong to you, and that you have no right to be a mother, are for many women a result of the way in which they are treated when they give birth in hospital. The disempowering of women during a major life transition is distressing not only at the time; it may have long term emotional effects. The memory of an unhappy birth experience affects a woman's attitude to future pregnancies and may remain with her for many years.

A woman who controls the space in which she gives birth, and who can therefore risk losing her self control, and surrender to the feelings welling up inside her during birth, is more likely to look back on the birth as a positive experience. She is less vulnerable to distress than one whose autonomy has been destroyed and who feels that she has been violated.

In an intimate, loving environment, the experience of birth can be empowering. Especially for any woman who is vulnerable to depression or violent mood swings, one with low self esteem, or who has suffered sexual abuse, birth can be healing. Childbirth is then an adventure in which you discover your own inner strength, joy in your body, and your capacity to give life and to open yourself in love.

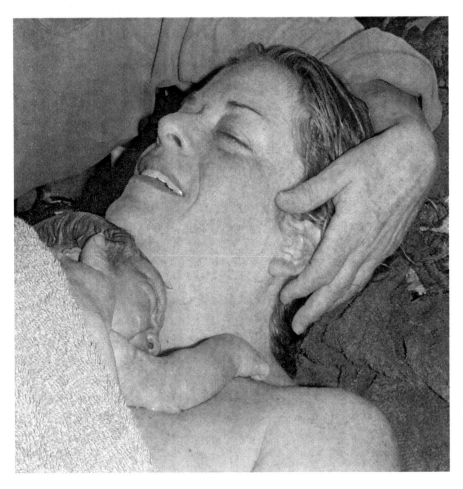

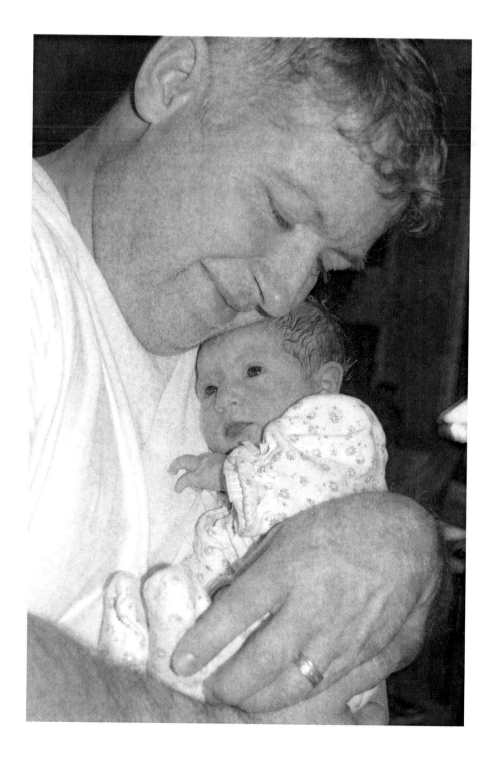

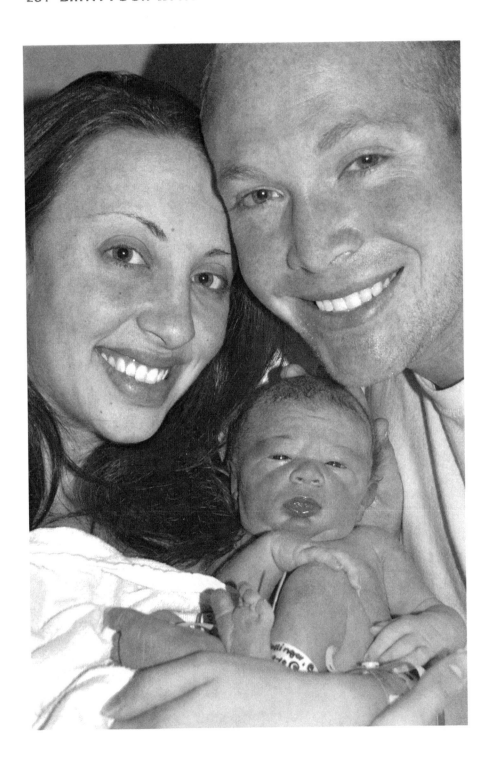

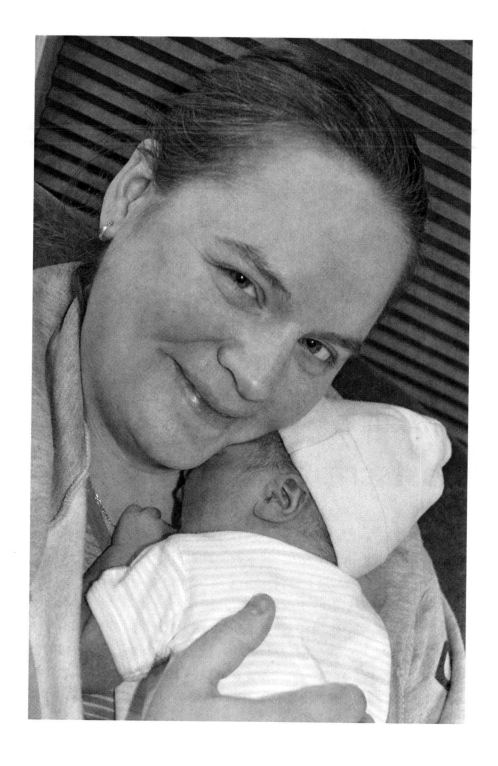

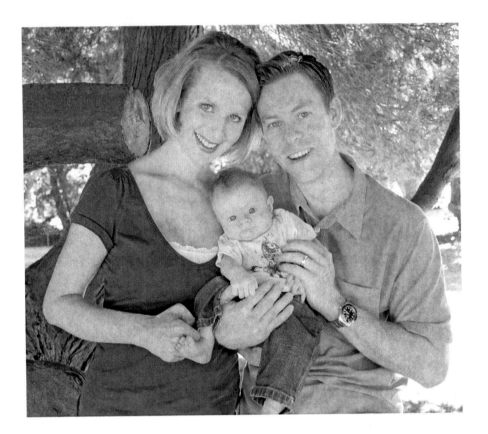

Postscript

Birth, like death, is a universal human experience that we share. It can be an interruption of life, a medical episode, a solitary trial of endurance, a surgical operation on a patient who relies entirely on the obstetric expertise of those caring for her, and a frightening process in which women are trapped by their biology. Or it can be lived through in beauty and dignity and as new life emerges cradled in love and caring, it can be a celebration of joy, which takes place in spite of pain—for the energy flooding through a woman's body in birth, although it brings pain as a side-effect, is life-enhancing and powerful.

Choosing their own birthplace—one in which they feel secure—creating a nest that meets the needs of the mother and her newborn, is something that all mammals do, unless, like animals in a zoo, they are in captivity.

> Women in our culture are effectively captive in childbirth. The zoo may be run on scientific principles, the keepers may be considerate... but captivity restrains and dictates behaviour.

Women in our post-industrial culture are effectively captive in childbirth. The zoo may be run on scientific principles, the keepers may be considerate and pride themselves on the good condition of their animals and the low mortality rate. Visiting times may be frequent and the zoo may be a friendly, welcoming place. In the confines of the cage there may be space to move about, and those in charge may have tried to replicate the natural habitat. Yet captivity restrains and dictates the behaviour of the captives.

At present saying 'no' to hospital, making an informed decision to give birth in a place of your own choosing, is for most of us the only way to reclaim the experience of childbirth for women.

> At present saying 'no' to hospital, making an informed decision to give birth in a place of your own choosing, is for most of us the only way to reclaim the experience of childbirth for women

There is a challenge facing the maternity services today over and above the basic requirement to make birth as safe as possible for mothers and babies. This challenge consists of two main issues. The first is to provide genuine choice. It must include the provision of a really good home birth service and, for those who prefer them, birth centres, midwifery-led units or GP units. The second important issue is to enable women giving birth in hospital to control the birthplace there, too, so that they are not merely at the receiving end of care, however kind and compassionate it may be.

When we affirm our freedom by making an informed choice, and select a place where we, not the doctors, are in control, we have an opportunity to rediscover in ourselves the power to give birth without any intervention, with the same confidence and spontaneity with which we breathe and move, and with the same love and passion with which we conceived the child who now enters the world.

Photo captions

You may like to look through the photos again to remind yourself of key points. Captions were not inserted alongside photos because the idea was not to spoil the flow of reading. Note that photos are copyright Patti Ramos, except when mentioned specially in the list below. For more photos by Patti, go to www.doulapattiramos.com

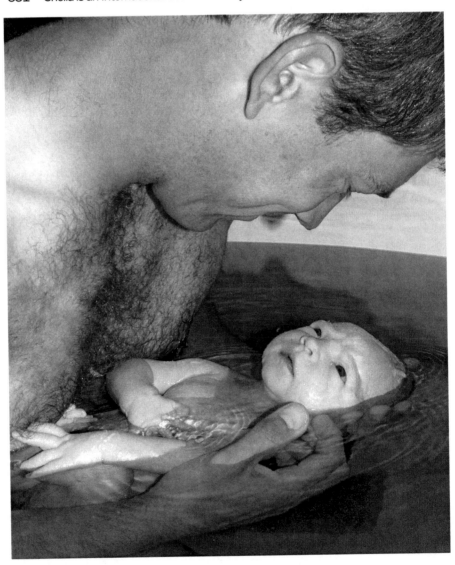

Useful contacts

Active Birth Centre – www.activebirthcentre.com

Tel: 020 7281 6760

Classes for mothers interested in active, physiological birth. Can put you in touch with local groups and supply birthing pools.

Active Birth Pools – www.activebirthpools.com

Tel: 0208 444 1411
Design and supply birthing pools.

AIMS (Association for Improvements in Maternity Services) – www.aims.org.uk

Helpline: 0300 365 0663
Support and information about parents' rights and choices. Provides information on complaints procedures.

Alexander Technique, Society for Teachers of (STAT) – www.stat.org.uk

Tel: 020 7482 5135
How to get help with physical co-ordination in pregnancy, birth and after.

Association of Breastfeeding Mothers – www.abm.me.uk

Helpline: 08444 122 949. Breastfeeding Help Line (National): 0300 100 0212
Support for breastfeeding.

Baby Milk Action – info.babymilkaction.org

Comments on the worldwide malpractices of the milk formula marketing companies.

Baby World – www.babyworld.co.uk

A strong political stance about the importance of breastfeeding.

Beautiful Birth Centre – www.gentlewater.co.uk

Tel: 01273 622001
Birthing pool hire.

Birth Choice – www.birthchoiceuk.com

UK maternity statistics and other useful information.

Birth Centres UK Network – www.birth.centres@ga.apc.org
How to find birth centre care.

BirthWorks – www.birthworks.co.uk
Tel: 0333 240 9710
Birthing pool hire.

Blue Lagoon Birth Pools – www.bluelagoonbirthpools.co.uk
Tel: 07949 016 877
Birthing pool hire.

BLISS – www.bliss.org.uk
Helpline: 0500 618140
Practical and emotional support for parents of premature babies.

The Breastfeeding Network – www.breastfeedingnetwork.org.uk
BfN supporterline: 0300 100 0210
For mothers and caregivers.

British Medical Journal – www.bmi.com
Highly respected refereed journal with a vast store of online articles including pregnancy, birth and breastfeeding.

The Cochrane Library – www.cochrane1.org
Cochrane reviews to read, under the topic: Pregnancy and Childbirth.

Doula UK – www.doula.org.uk
Tel: 0871 433 3103
Information about birth and postnatal doulas working in your area.

Down's Syndrome Association – www.downs-syndrome.org.uk
Tel: 0845 230 0372
For help if you are likely to have or already have a Down's baby.

Gingerbread – www.gingerbread.org.uk
Tel: 0808 802 0925
Information on lone parenting.

The Good Birth Company – www.thegoodbirth.co.uk
Birthing pool hire (inflatable birthing pools).

Group B Strep Support – www.gbss.org.uk
Tel: 01444 416176
Useful information for women who have been diagnosed as Strep B positive.

Home Birth Reference Site – www.homebirth.org.uk
Information on home birth, including a list of home birth support groups in the UK.

Independent Midwives UK – www.independentmidwives.org.uk
Tel: 0845 460 0105 (answer machine)
Association for independent midwives. Can provide list of independent midwives in your area, experienced in home birth.

Irish Childbirth Trust – www.cuidiu.com
Tel: Dublin (01) 8724501
The NCT in Ireland.

La Leche League Great Britain – www.laleche.org.uk
Tel: 0845 456 1855
Support and information for pregnant women and breastfeeding mothers. Network of informal support groups.

Maternity Action – www.maternityaction.org.uk
Tel: 020 7253 2288
Organisation which challenges inequality and promotes well-being.

Meet-a-Mum Association (MAMA) – www.mama.co.uk
Helpline: 0845 120 3746
Support for mothers who feel lonely, isolated or depressed. Can put you in touch with other mothers in a similar situation.

Midirs (Midwives Information and Resource Service) – www.midirs.org
Vast resources for midwives. Important reading for student midwives.

Midirs Informed Choice Leaflets – www.choicesforbirth.org
Excellent leaflets, by birth topic, for professionals and mothers.

Mumsnet – www.mumsnet.com

A lively webpage, discusses and presents mothers' views in a political context.

Natal Hypotherapy – www.natalhypnotherapy.co.uk

Self hypnosis CDs, books and workshops.

National Childbirth Trust (NCT) – www.nct.org.uk

Enquiries: 0300 330 0770. Breastfeeding helpline: 0300 330 0771
Pregnancy and Birth helpline: 0300 330 0772. Postnatal helpline: 0300 330 0773
Information and support for all aspects of pregnancy and birth. Antenatal classes and network of informal postnatal groups.

Patients Association – www.patients-association.org.uk

Helpline: 0845 608 4455
Useful if you want to follow up a complaint about care.

Association of Radical Midwives – www.midwifery.org.uk

Helpline: 01865 248159
Place to find midwife care that supports home birth and birth in a birth centre.

Second Nature Birthing – www.naturalchildbirth.co.uk

HypnoBirthing.

Sheila Kitzinger's website – www.sheilakitzinger.com

Information and articles on various aspects of birth, as well as details about Sheila's work—particularly the Birth Crisis Network and workshops.

Stillbirth and Neonatal Death Society (SANDS) – www.uk-sands.org

Helpline: 020 7438 5881
Support and information for bereaved parents.

Twins and Multiples Births Association (TAMBA) – www.tamba.org.uk

Tel: 01483 304 442. Twinline: 0800 138 0509
Encouragement and support for parents of twins or more.

VBAC Information and Support – www.vbac.org.uk

Tel: 01243 868440
Support for women who are planning to have a vaginal birth after one or more previous caesareans.

References

Why give birth at home or in a birth centre?

1   Doering S, Entwistle D. Preparation during pregnancy and ability to cope with labor and delivery. *American Journal of Orthopsychiatry*, 1975; 45:825-837

2   Norr K, Block C, Charles A, et al. Explaining pain and enjoyment in childbirth, *Journal of Health and Social Behaviour*, 1977; 10:260-275

3   Doering S, Entwistle D, Quinlan D. Modeling the quality of women's birth experience, *Journal of Health and Social Behaviour*, 1980; 21:12-21

4   Entwistle D, Doering S. *The First Birth,* John Hopkins University Press, Baltimore, 1981

5   Romito P. Unhappiness after childbirth, edited by Chalmers I, Enkin M, Keirse M, *Effective Care in Pregnancy and Childbirth*, 1989; 2:1433-1446

6   Kitzinger J. Labour relations: Midwives and doctors on the ward, in Garcia J, Kilpatrick R, Richards M, Eds. *The Politics of Maternity Care*, Clarendon Press, Oxford, 1990, pp.149-162

7   Kitzinger S. Childbirth and violence against women, in Roberts H, ed. *Women's Health Matters,* Routledge, London, 1991; Kitzinger S. *Some Women's Experiences of Epidurals*, National Childbirth Trust, London, 1987.

Questioning hospital practices

1   Morse J M, Park C. Home birth and hospital deliveries: A comparison of the perceived painfulness of parturition, *Research in Nursing & Health*, 1988; 11:175-181.

2   Lowe N K. Individual variation in childbirth pain, *Journal of Psychosomatic Research,* 1987; 20: 212-221; Fridh G, Kopare T, Gaston-Jophansson F, et al. Factors associated with more intense labor pain. *Research in Nursing and Health*, 1988; 11:117-124.

3   Morse J M, Park C, *op cit.*; Fridh G, Kopare T, Gaston-Jophansson F, et al, *op cit.*

4   Fridh G, Kopare T, Gaston-Jophansson F, et al, *op cit.*

5   Simkin P. Stress, pain and catecholamines in labor: part 1, a review, *Birth*, 1986; 13:4:227-233.

6   Association of Anaesthetists. *Report on Obstetric Services*, London, 1988.

7   Chamberlain G, Zander L. Induction. *British Medical Journal*, 1999; 318:995-997.

8   Kitzinger S. *Some Women's Experiences of Induced Labour*, National Childbirth Trust, London, 1975.

9   O'Driscoll K, Meagher D. Active management of labour. Saunders W, ed. *Clinical and Obstetric Gynaecology (supplement 1)*, 1980.

10   O'Driscoll K, Meagher D, *op cit.*

11   O'Driscoll K, Meagher D, *op cit.*

12   O'Driscoll K, Meagher D, *op cit.*

13   Taylor R, Taylor M. Letter to the *Lancet*, 1988; 1:8581:352.

14   Nielson P, Stigsby B, Nickelson C, et al. Intra- and inter-observer variability in the assessment of intrapartum cardiotocograms, *Acta Obstetrica et Gynecologia Scandinavica*, 1987; 66:421-424.

15   Grant A. Monitoring the fetus during labour. Chalmers I, Enkin M, Keirse M, eds. *Effective Care in Pregnancy and Childbirth*, Oxford University Press, Oxford, 1989; 2:846-882.

16   Macdonald D, Grant A, Sheridan-Pereira M, et al. The Dublin randomized trial of intrapartum fetal heart rate monitoring, *American Journal of Obstetrics and Gynecology*, 1985; 152:524-539.

17   Grant, A. The relationship between obstetrically preventable intrapartum asphyxia, abnormal neonatal neurological signs and subsequent motor impairment in babies born at or after term; Kubli F, Patel N, Schmidt W, et al, eds. *Perinatal Events and Brain Damage in Surviving Children*, Springer Verlag, Berlin, 1987.

18   Amato J. Fetal heart-rate monitoring, *American Journal of Obstetrics and Gynecology*, 1983; 147:967-969.

19   Visser G, Goodman J, Dawes G. Problems with ultrasonic fetal heart-rate monitor, *Lancet,* 1:707-708.

20   Sharp D, Couriel J. Penetration of the subarachnoid space by fetal scalp electrode, *British Medical Journal*, 1985; 291:1169.

21   D'Douza S. Fetal scalp damage and neonatal jaundice: A risk of fetal scalp electrode monitoring, *International Journal of Obstetrics and Gynecology*, 1982; 2:161-164.

22   Enkin M. Labour and delivery following previous caesarean section. Chalmers I, Enkin M, Keirse M, eds. *Effective Care in Pregnancy and Childbirth*, Oxford University Press, 1989; 2:1196-1217.

23   Findley I, Chamberlain G. ABC of Labour Care: Relief of Pain, *British Medical Journal,* 1999; 318:927-930.

24   Kitzinger S. Perceptions of pain in home and hospital birth. Paper given at the International Congress of Psychosomatic Obstetrics and Gynaecology, Amsterdam, 1989.

25   Garcia J, Garforth S, Ayers S. Midwives confined? Labour ward policies and routines, *Research and the Midwife Conference Proceedings*, University of Manchester, 1986; 74-78.

26   Cohen W. Influence and the duration of second stage labor on perinatal outcome and puerperal morbidity, *Obstetrics and Gynecology*, 1977; 49:266-269.

27   Caldeyro-Barcia R. The influence of maternal bearing-down efforts during second stage on fetal wellbeing, *Birth and the Family Journal*, 1979; 6:17-21.

28   Thacker S, Banta H. Benefits and risks of episiotomy: An interpretive review of the English language literature, 1860-1980, *Obstetrical and Gynecological Survey*, 1983; 38:322-338.

29   Sleep J, Grant A, Garcia J, et al. West Berkshire perineal management trial, *British Medical Journal*, 1984; 289:587-590; Harrison R, Brennan M, North P, et al. Is routine episiotomy necessary? *British Medical Journal,*

1984; 288:1971-1975; Sleep J, Grant A. West Berkshire perineal management trial: Three year follow-up, *British Medical Journal*, 1987; 295:749-751.

30 Sleep J, Grant A, Garcia J, *op cit*.; Harrison R, Brennan M, North P. *op cit*.

31 Kitzinger S, Simkin P. *Episiotomy and the Second Stage of Labor*. Pennypress Inc. Seattle, 1990.

32 Kitzinger S, Walters R. *Some Women's Experiences of Episiotomy*, National Childbirth Trust, London, 1981.

33 Davis E. *Heart and Hands*, Celestial Arts, California, 1981; Flint C. *Sensitive Midwifery*, Heinemann, London, 1986; 101-102.

34 Neu H. The crisis in antibiotic resistance, *Science*, 1992; 257:1064-73.

35 Weiner J. *The Beak of the Finch*, Vintage Books, New York, 1995; 257.

36 Cordero L, Hon E. Neonatal bradychardia following nasopharyngeal stimulation, *Journal of Pediatrics*, 1971; 78:441-447.

37 Tyson J, Silverman W, Reisch J. Immediate care of the newborn infant in Chalmers I, Enkin M, Keirse M, eds. *Effective Care in Pregnancy and Childbirth*, 1989; 2:1293-1312.

38 Cordero L, Hon E, *op cit*.; Widstrom A, RansjoArvidson A, Christeosson K, et al. Gastric suction in healthy newborn infants: Effects on circulation and developing feeding behaviour, *Acta Paediatrica Scandinavica*, 1987; 76:566-572.

39 Wahlberg V, Lundh W, Winberg J. Reconsideration of Crede prophylaxis III: Effects of silver nitrate prophylaxis on visual alertness in neonates, *Acta Paediatrica Scandinavica*, 1982; 295 (supplement): 43-48; Wahlberg V, Lundh W, Winberg J. Reconsideration of Crede prophylaxis IV: Effects of silver nitrate prophylaxis on mother infant relationship, *Acta Paediatrica Scandinavica*, 1982; 295 (supplement): 49-57; Wahlberg V, Lundh W, Winberg J. Reconsideration of Crede prophylaxis V: Long-term influences on conjunctival secretion, infant behaviour, breastfeeding and maternal feelings. A descriptive study, *Acta Paediatrica Scandinavica*, 1982; 295 (supplement): 59-67.

40 Rothenberg R. Ophthalmia neonatorum due to Neisseria gonorrhoeae: Prevention and treatment, *Sexually Transmitted Diseases,* 1979; 6 (supplement): 187-1990.

41 Hammerschlag M, Chandler J, Alexander R, et al. Erythromycin ointment for ocular prophylaxis of neonatal chlamydial infection, *Journal of the American Medical Association,* 1980; 244:2291-2293.

42 World Health Organization, 1985.

43 Waterstone M, Bewley, Wolfe C. Incidence and predictors of sever obstetric morbidity case-control study, *British Medical Journal,* 2001; 322:1089-1093.

44 Murphy D. Commentary: Obstetric morbidity data and the need to evaluate thromboembolic disease, *British Medical Journal,* 2001; 322:1093-1094.

Understanding safety

1 Wickham S. Reflecting on risk assessment, *Essentially MIDIRS,* 2010; 1:2:50-51.

2 Mahmood T, Campbell D, Wilson A. Maternal height, shoe size, and outcome of labour in white primigravidas: A prospective anthropometric study, *British Medical Journal,* 1988; 297:515-517.

3 Campbell R, Macfarlane A. Recent debate on the place of birth. Garcia J, Kilpatrick R, Richards M, eds. *The Politics of Maternity Care,* Oxford University Press, Oxford, 1990; 217-237.

4 Social Security Committee. *Perinatal and Neonatal Mortality,* (second report), HMSO, London, 1980.

5 Bragg F, Cromwell DA, Edozien LC, *et al.* Variation in rates of caesarean section among English NHS Trusts after accounting for natural and clinical risk: cross sectional study, BMJ 2010;341:c5065

6 Woodcock H, Read A, Moore D, et al. Planned home-births in Western Australia 1981-1987: A descriptive study, *Medical Journal of Australia,* 1990; 153:672-678.

7   Tew M. *Safer Childbirth*, Chapman & Hall, London, 1990.

8   Olsen O. Meta-analysis of the Safety of Home Birth, *Birth*, 1997; 24:1:4-13.

9   Chamberlain G, Wraight A, Crowley P. *Home Birth: The Report of the 1994 Confidential Enquiry by the National Birthday Trust Fund*, Parthenon, London, 1997.

10 Wax J, Lucas F, Lamont M, et al. Maternal and newborn outcomes in planned home birth vs planned hospital births: a metaanalysis. *American Journal of Obstetrics and Gynecology*. 2010; 203:3:243.e1-243.e8. Accessed 5 October 2010. Available at http://www.ajog.org/article/S0002-9378%2810%2900671-X.

11 Editors. Home birth - proceed with caution. *The Lancet*. July 2010; 376:9738;303. doi:10.1016/S0140-6736(10)61165-8

12 Warwick C. Quote in Randeep Ramesh (6 August 2010) "Midwives attack hysteria over home births". The Guardian. Accessed 5 October 2010. Available at http://www.guardian.co.uk/lifeandstyle/2010/aug/16/homebirths-midwives-hospital-baby; Gyte G, Newburn, M and Macfarlane, Critical Appraisal, Essentially MIDIRS October 2010 20-22

13 Wax J, Lucas F, Lamont M, et al. Maternal and newborn outcomes in planned home birth vs planned hospital births: a metaanalysis. *op cit*.

14 Pang JW, Heffelfinger JD, Huang GJ, et al. Outcomes of planned home births in Washington State: 1989—1996. *Obstet Gynecol* 2002; 100: 253-259.

15 Vedam S. Home birth versus hospital birth: questioning the quality of evidence on safety. *Birth* 2003; 30: 57-63.

16 Gyte G, Newburn M, Macfarlane A. Critique of a meta-analysis by Wax and colleagues which has claimed that there is a three times greater risk of neonatal death among babies without congenital anomalies planned to be born at home. NCT. 7 July 2010. Accessed 5 October 2010. Available at http://www.nct.org.uk/about-us/what-we-do/policy/choiceofplaceofbirth.

17 CIMS Responds to Skewed Article on Homebirth. Coalition for Improving Maternity Services, press release 9th July 2010. Accessed 5 October

2010. Available at http://www.motherfriendly.org/
CIMSResponseToSkewedData.php.

18   Klein M quoted in CIMS Responds to Skewed Article on Homebirth. *op cit.*

19   Wright J. Alcohol and drug abuse in pregnancy, *Medicine International,*
1983; 35:1630-1631.

20   Calandra C, Abell D, Beiseher N. Maternal obesity in pregnancy, *Obstetrics
and Gynecology,* 1981; 57:8-12; Garbakiak J, Richter M, Miller S, et al.
Maternal weight and pregnancy complications, *American Journal of
Obstetrics and Gynecology,* 1985; 152:238-245.

21   Garbakiak J, et al, *op cit.*

22   Chamberlain G, et al, *op cit.*; James D, Stirrat G, eds. *Pregnancy and Risk:
The Basis for Rational Management,* John Wiley & Sons, Chichester,
1988.

23   Hofmeyr G. Breech presentation and abnormal lie in late pregnancy,
Chalmers I, Enkin M, Keirse M, eds. *Effective Care in Pregnancy and
Childbirth,* Oxford University Press, Oxford, 1989; 1:635-666.

24   Hughey M. Fetal position during pregnancy, *American Journal of
Obstetrics and Gynecology,* 1985; 153:885-886.

25   Westgren M, Edvall H, Nordstrom F, et al. Spontaneous cephalic version of
breech presentation in the late trimester, *British Journal of Obstetrics and
Gynaecology,* 1985; 92:19-22.

26   Bakketeig L, Hoffman J. Epidemiology of preterm birth: Results from a
longitudinal study of births in Norway, Elder M, Hendricks, C, eds.
Butterworth's International Medical Review, Preterm Labour, London,
1981; 17-40.

27   Salzmann B. Rupture of low segment cesarean section, *American Journal
of Obstetrics and Gynecology,* 1964; 23:460-466.

28   Beard R, Lowy C. The British survey of diabetic pregnancies, *British
Journal of Obstetrics and Gynaecology,* 1986; 89:78326.

29   James D, Stirrat G, eds. *op cit.*

30 De Swiet M. Preexisting medical diseases, Chamberlain G, Lumley J, eds. *Pregnancy Care: A Manual for Practice,* John Wiley & Sons, Chichester, 1986; 69-111.

31 Bird C. The premenopausal gravida, *Journal of Reproductive Medicine,* 1971; 6:48-50.

32 Kirz D, Dorchester W, Freeman R. Advanced maternal age, *American Journal of Obstetrics and Gynecology,* 1985; 152:1:7-12.

33 Cario G, Fray R, Morris N. The obstetric performance of the elderly primigravida, *British Journal of Obstetrics and Gynaecology,* 1985; 54:237-240.

34 Taylor D, et al. Do pregnancy complications contribute to neurodevelopmental disability? Lancet, 1985; 1:713-716.

35 Steer P. Risks in labour. James D, Stirrat G, eds. *Pregnancy and Risk,* 1988; 6:105-137.

Making arrangements

1 Saunders D, et al. *Evaluation of the Edgware Birth Centre,* North Thames Perinatal Public Health, London, 2000.

2 Feldman E, Hurst M. A comparison of hospital and birth center settings, *Birth,* 1987; 18-24.

3 Lumley J, Davey B. Do hospitals with family-centered maternity care policies have lower intervention rates? *Birth,* 1987; 132-134.

4 Klein M, et al. Care in a birth room versus a conventional setting: A controlled trial, *Canadian Medical Association Journal,* 1984; 131:1461-1466.

5 Rosenblatt K, Reinken J, Shoemack P. Is obstetrics safe in small hospitals? Evidence from New Zealand's regionalized perinatal system, *Lancet,* 1985; 2:429-432.

6 Mugford M, Stilwell J. Maternity services: How well have they done and could they do better? *Health Care,* Policy Journals, 1986.

7   *Human Rights Act*, Stationery Office, London, 1998.

8   McCall Smith A. Obtaining consent for examination and treatment, *British Medical Journal,* 2001; 322:811-812.

Your midwife

1   Hood S. Midwifery in some European countries. Van Hall E, Everaerd W, eds. *op cit.*

2   Barrington E. Birth stories and midwives' musings, *Midwifery is Catching,* 1985; 101.

3   Kirkham M. A feminist perspective in midwifery, Webb C, ed. *Feminist Practice in Women's Healthcare,* John Wiley & Sons, Chichester, 1986.

Getting ready

1   Office of Population Censuses and Surveys. *Mortality Statistics, Perinatal and Infant: Social and Biological Factors,* series DH3, HMSO, London, 1986; 17.

2   Serkin M, Porte J, Monheit A. *The relationship of antepartum pelvic examinations to the incidence of premature rupture of the membranes, maternal infection, and cesarean section.* Paper given at the Scientific Session of Annual Clinical Meeting of American College of Obstetricians and Gynecologists, May 1988.

3   Pearch J, Campbell S. A comparison of symphysis-fundal height and ultrasound screening tests for light-for-gestational age infants, *British Journal of Obstetrics and Gynaecology,* 1987; 94:100-104.

4   Alexander S, et al. Biochemical assessment of fetal well-being, Chalmers I, Enkin M, Keirse M, eds. *Effective Care in Pregnancy and Childbirth,* 1989; 1:455-476.

5   Mohide P, Keirse M. Biophysical assessment of fetal well-being, Chalmers I, Enkin M, Keirse M, eds. *op cit.* 1989; 1:455-476.

6   Robinson M. Salt in pregnancy, *Lancet,* 1958; 1:178-181.

7   Rush D. Effects of changes in protein and calorie intake during pregnancy on the growth of the human fetus, Chalmers I, Enkin M, Keirse M, eds. *op cit.* 255-280.

8   McIntyre A. *Herbs for Pregnancy and Childbirth,* Sheldon, London, 1988.

9   Hemminki E, Starfield B. Routine administration of iron and vitamins during pregnancy: Review of controlled clinical trials, *British Journal of Obstetrics and Gynaecology,* 1985; 85:404-410.

10   Alexander S, et al, *op cit.*

11   Burns E, Blamey S, Ersser A, et al. *The use of aromatherapy in intrapartum midwifery practice: An evaluative study,* Oxford Centre for Health Care Research and Development, Oxford Brookes University, 1999.

12   Burns E, Kitzinger S. *Midwifery Guidelines for Use of Water in Labour,* School of Health and Social Care, Oxford Brookes University, 3rd edition, 2010.

13   Kitzinger S. *Politics of Birth,* Elsevier, Oxford, 2005; 123-134.

Your birth partner

1   Richards M, Dunn J, Antonis B. Caretaking in the first year of life: The role of fathers' and mothers' social isolation, *Child Care Health Development,* 1977; 3:23-36.

2   Berry L. Realistic expectation of the labor coach, *Journal of Obstetric Gynecological and Neonatal Nursing,* 1988; 17:5:354-355.

3   Perez P, Snedeker C. Why parents need professional labor support, *Special Women,* Pennypress Inc. Seattle, 1990.

4   Kitzinger S. *Pregnancy and Childbirth: Choices and Challenges,* Dorling Kindersley, London, revised 2008.

Sharing the experience

1   Donnison J. *Midwives and Medical Men,* Heinemann, London, 1990.

2   Pollock L. *A Lasting Relationship: Parents and Children over Three Centuries,* Fourth Estate, London, 1987.

3   Kitzinger S. *Rediscovering Birth*, Pinter and Martin, London, 2010.

4   Mason J, quoting Miles L. Pioneer Questionnaires (Health) SX-2, in Midwifery in Canada, Kitzinger S, ed. *The Midwife Challenge,* Pandora, London, 1988.

5   Mason J, quoting Miles L, *op cit.*

6   Benoit C. Midwives and healers: The Newfoundland experience, *Health Sharing,* 1983; 22-25.

7   Benoit C, *op cit.*

8   Klaus M, Kennell J, Robertson S, et al. Effects of social support during parturition on maternal-infant morbidity, *British Medical Journal,* 1986; 293:585-587.

9   Hosnett F, Osborn R. A randomized trial of the effects of monitrice support during labor: Mothers' views two to four weeks postpartum, *Birth,* 1989; 16:4:177-184.

10 Flint C. *Sensitive Midwifery,* Heinemann, London, 1986.

11 Kitzinger S. *Being Born,* Dorling Kindersley, London, 1986.

Meeting challenges

1   Rossavik L. *Obstetrics and Gynecology,* 1989; 73:2:243-249.

2   Yudkin P, Wood L, Redman C. Rise of unexplained stillbirth at different gestational stages, *Lancet,* 1987; 1192-1194.

3   Lamont R. Management of preterm labour, *Hospital Update,* 1986; 487-490, 492-493.

4   Salmon Y. Cervical ripening by breast stimulation, *Obstetrics and*

Gynecology, 1986; 67:1:21-24; Curtis P. Uterine responses to three techniques of breast stimulation, *Obstetrics and Gynecology,* 1986; 67:1:22-28; Curtis F. Prepartum and intrapartum breast stimulation in obstetrics, *Journal of Reproductive Medicine,* 1986; 31:4:228-230.

5 Sinquefield G. Midwifery management of premature rupture of the membranes at term, *Journal of Nurse Midwifery,* 1985; 30:4:242-244.

6 Lenihan J. The relationship of antepartum pelvic examinations to premature rupture of the membranes, *Obstetrics and Gynecology,* 1984; 63:33-37.

7 Davis E. *Heart and Hands,* Celestial Arts, California, 1987.

8 Butler N, Bonham D. *Perinatal Mortality,* Churchill Livingstone, Edinburgh, 1963.

9 McKay S. How worthwhile are membrane stripping and amniotomy? *Contemporary Obstetrics and Gynecology,* 1983; 173-176,178-181,184.

10 Newton N, Foshea D, Newton M. Experimental inhibition of labor through environmental disturbance, *Obstetrics and Gynecology,* 1966; 67:371-377.

11 Salar G, et al. Effect of transcutaneous electrotherapy on cerebro spinal fluid beta-endorphin content in patients without pain problems, *Pain,* 1981; 10:169-172; Polden M. Transcutaneous nerve stimulation in labour and post-Caesarean section, *Physiotherapy,* 71:8:350-353.

12 Harrison R, et al. Pain relief in labour using transcutaneous electrical nerve stimulation (TENS), *British Journal of Obstetrics and Gynaecology, 1986; 93:7:739, 746.*

13 Flint C, *op cit.*

14 Davis E, *op cit.*

15 Simkin P. *The Birth Partner,* Harvard Common Press, 1989.

16 Gaskin I. Ask the midwives, *The Practicing Midwife,* 1982; 1:15.

17 Lawrence H. Breathing for labour, *Journal of Association of Chartered Physiotherapists and Obstetrics in Gynaecology,* 1988; 60:2:21-23.

18 Broach J, Newton N. Food and beverages in labor. Part 1: Cross-cultural and historical practices. Part 2: The effects of cessation of oral intake during labor, *Birth,* 1988; 2:15.

19 Davis E, *op cit.*

20 Newton N, Foshea D, Newton M, *op cit.*

21 Sleep J, Roberts J, Chalmers I. Care during the second stage of labour, Enkin M, Keirse M, Neilson J, et al. eds. *A Guide to Effective Care in Pregnancy and Childbirth,* Oxford University Press, Oxford, 3rd edition 2000.

22 Cronk M, Flint C. *Community Midwifery: A Practical Guide,* Heinemann, London, 1989.

23 Gaskin I. *Spiritual Midwifery,* Book Publishing Company, Tennessee, 1978.

24 Stein A. Breech delivery: A co-operative nurse-midwifery medical management approach, *Journal of Nurse-midwifery,* 1986; 31:2:93-97.

25 Odent M. *Birth Reborn,* Random House, New York, 1984.

26 Russell J. The rationale of primitive delivery positions, *British Journal of Obstetrics and Gynaecology,* 1982; 89:712-715.

27 Sleep J, Roberts J, Chalmers I, *op cit.*

28 O'Leary J, Gunn D. Options for shoulder dystocia: cephalic replacement, *Contemporary Obstetrics and Gynecology,* 1986; 27:157.

29 Gaskin I. Shoulder dystocia: Controversies in management, *Birth Gazette,* 1988; 5:1:14-17.

30 Flint C, *op cit.*

31 Davis E, *op cit.*

32 Davis E, *op cit.*

33 Davis E, *op cit.*

34 Davis E, *op cit.*

Enjoying your babymoon

1   Leavitt J. *Brought to Bed: Childbearing in America 1750-1950,* Oxford University Press, New York, 1986.

2   Kitzinger S. *Rediscovering Birth*, Pinter and Martin, London, 2010.

3   Winnicott D, *The Child, the Family, and the Outside World,* Penguin, London, 1964.

4   Garforth S, Garcia J. Breastfeeding policies and practice - 'no wonder they get confused', *Midwifery,* 1989; 5:2:75-83.

5   Garforth S, Garcia J, *op cit.*

6   Kitzinger S. *The New Good Birth Guide*, Penguin, London, 1983.

7   Woolridge M. *Right from the start - establishing breastfeeding,* Symposium on Caring for the Breastfeeding Mother, Kings Fund Centre, London, 1988.

8   Office of Population, Censuses and Surveys, Social Security Division. *Infant Feeding,* HMSO, London, 1988.

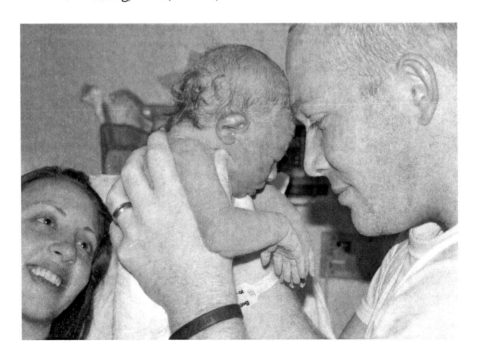

9   Kitzinger S. *Breastfeeding Your Baby,* Dorling Kindersley, London, 1988.

10 Pitt B. Atypical depression following childbirth, *British Journal of Psychiatry,* 1968; 114:1325-1335.

11 Stein A, et al. Social adversity and perinatal complications: Their relationship to postnatal depression, *British Medical Journal,* 1989; 290.

12 Kitzinger S. *Birth Crisis,* Routledge, Abingdon, 2006.

13 Oakley A. *Women Confined,* Martin Robertson, Oxford, 1980.

14 Alfonso D. *Impact of Cesarean Childbirth,* Davis, Philadelphia, 1981; Bradley C, et al. A prospective study of mothers' attitudes and feelings following cesarean and vaginal births, *Birth,* 1983; 10:79-83; Garel M, et al. Psychological consequences of caesarean childbirth in primiparas, *Journal of Psychosomatic Obstetrics and Gynaecology,* 1987; 6:197-209.

15 Thune-Larsen K, Mailer Pedersen K. Childbirth experience and postpartum emotional disturbance, *Journal of Reproductive and Infant Psychology,* 1988; 6:229-240.

16 Kitzinger S. Birth and violence against women, in Roberts H. ed. *Women's Health Matters,* Routledge, London. 1992; Kitzinger S. *The Year After Childbirth,* Oxford University Press, Oxford, 1994.

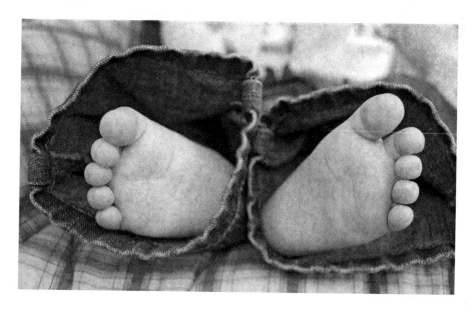

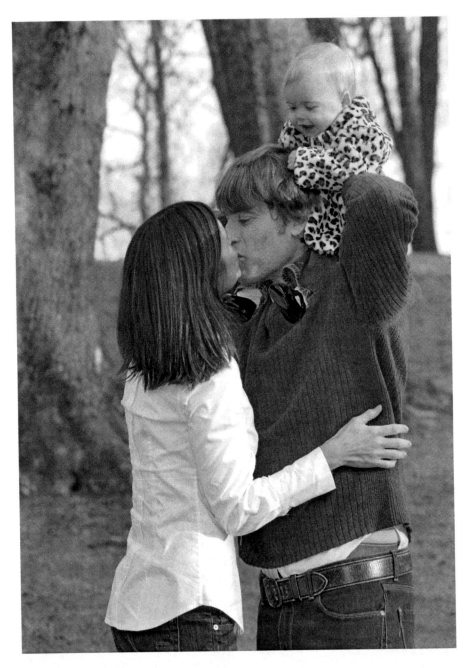

A child learns about positive relationships by witnessing them
and being drawn into a circle of love

Index

Quick reference index

Q&A boxes

Questions you may be wondering about

Birth partner tips

Also available...

Other books to help you prepare, if you're pregnant...

Birth: Countdown to Optimal: information and inspiration for pregnant women—by Sylvie Donna

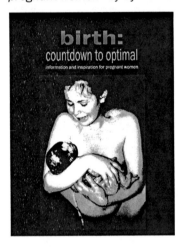

Birthing Normally After a Caesarean or Two: exploring reasons and practicalities for VBAC—by Hélène Vadeboncoeur

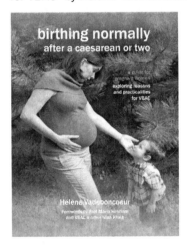

Birth Pain: Power to Transform: a guide for pregnant women—by Verena Schmid

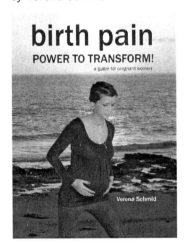

Surprising, Inspiring Birth: accounts of birth to inform, amuse and reassure—by Sylvie Donna (ed)

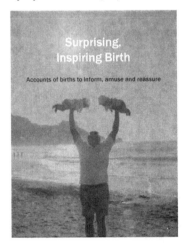

Books your caregivers may find useful...

Optimal Birth: What, Why & How—
a reflective narrative approach based
*on research evidence—*by Sylvie Donna

Promoting Normal Birth: Research,
Reflections & Guidelines—
an international collaboration

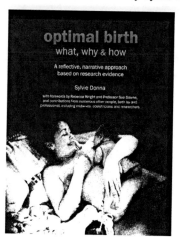

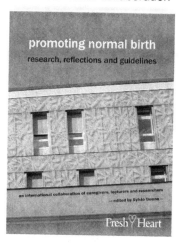

Birth Pain: Explaining sensations,
exploring possibilities—
by Verena Schmid

Welcoming Baby: a reflective guide
for midwives [on neonatal care]—
by Debby Gould

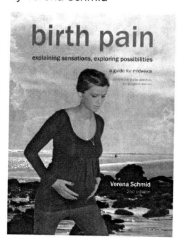

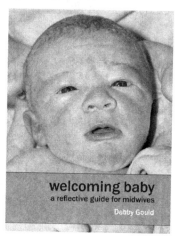

See the website for info and prices. All books are also available from Amazon.

www.freshheartpublishing.co.uk

About the author

A social anthropologist specialising in childbirth, Sheila Kitzinger has done fieldwork on birth in Jamaica, South Africa, Mexico, New Zealand (learning from the Maoris), Italy and Eastern European countries. She has also worked as a lecturer, birth educator and activist.

She lectures for universities and gives talks for birth and midwifery organisations around the world. She is also an examiner of academic theses in the UK and Australia and has been an Honorary Professor of Midwifery at Thames Valley University since 1994.

Becoming increasingly aware over the years of the problems that many women face, Sheila set up the Birth Crisis Network so as to support people who are distressed after traumatic births. She runs training days for midwives, doctors, doulas, therapists and birth educators, and has worked with the NCT (the National Childbirth Trust) since its foundation. She also created a teacher training scheme and set up many research projects on women's experiences, working in collaboration with the NCT and contributed textual material for birth exhibitions at the Smithsonian, Washington and Natural Science museums. As a board member of MIDIRS (the research organisation which provides information to midwives and pregnant women), as a regular columnist for the journal *Birth* (published by Blackwell Science), and as a regular contributor of articles to newspapers and magazines, Sheila continues to promote the best interests of pregnant women and their babies.

Her campaigning work has focused on issues such as the need for women to be able to make their own birth plans, induction of labour, hospital birth and episiotomy, and she works with lawyers on human rights issues relevant to pregnant women, including those who are in prison or seeking asylum in the UK. Sheila is a strong believer that all women who are not at high risk—and that is most women—should have the choice of a home birth. For many years she has campaigned to promote women's right to make their own informed decisions about childbirth, whether they feel most comfortable giving birth at home, in a hospital or at a birth centre. This book is part of her work to help women become aware of their options.

In fact, Sheila has been a prolific writer for many years and her work has now been published in 23 languages. Her books include: *The Politics of Birth* (Elsevier, 2005), *The New Pregnancy and Childbirth* (Dorling Kindersley, 2011), *Rediscovering Birth* (Pinter & Martin, 2011) and *Birth Crisis* (Routledge, 2006).

Unsurprisingly, perhaps, her books have received many awards, including the Horn Book Award and The Times Literary Award, and she was awarded an MBE for services in childbirth education. Since 2006, she has even had her portrait in the National Portrait Gallery in London—as one of the individuals who have made a major contribution to health in the UK.

To sum up, when you read this book, you can be certain that you're reading the words of a true expert. Not only has Sheila given birth to five babies herself, she has also worked with many other women, and midwives too, so she has a very broad perspective of the personal and practical challenges you might face when you plan your own birth—wherever you choose that to be.

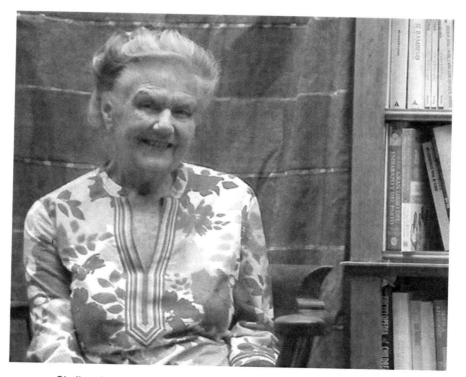

Sheila relaxing at home, alongside a few of her several hundred books

CPSIA information can be obtained at www.ICGtesting.com
Printed in the USA
LVOW131507221211

260734LV00005B/99/P